Smart Health Choices

Making sense of health advice

Professor Les Irwig
Judy Irwig
Dr Lyndal Trevena
Melissa Sweet

Cartoons by Ron Tandberg

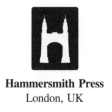

Hammersmith Press
London, UK

First published in 2008 by Hammersmith Press Limited
496 Fulham Palace Road, London SW6 6JD, UK
www.hammersmithpress.co.uk

Disclaimer
Whilst the advice and information in this book are believed to be true and accurate at the date of going to press, neither the author nor the publisher can accept any legal responsibility or liability for any errors or omissions that may be made.

British Library Cataloguing in Publication Data: A CIP record of this book is available from the British Library.

ISBN 978-1-905140-17-6

Commissioning Editor: Georgina Bentliff
Copy editing by Jane Sugarman
Designed by Julie Bennett
Production by Helen Whitehorn, Pathmedia
Typeset by Phoenix Photosetting, Chatham, Kent, UK
Printed and bound by TJ International Ltd, Padstow, Cornwall, UK
Cover image: © Photolibrary Group

Smart Health Choices

Please return / renew by date shown.
You can renew it at:
norlink.norfolk.gov.uk
or by telephone: 0344 800 8006
Please have your library card & PIN ready

NORFOLK COUNTY LIBRARY
WITHDRAWN FOR SALE

NORFOLK LIBRARY
AND INFORMATION SERVICE

In loving memory of Andre Joffe
1964–1999
He touched the lives of so many people
In so many extraordinary ways

Contents

Part V: Improving your healthcare

Part VI: Testing your skill

About the authors

Les Irwig MB BCH, PhD is an internationally renowned expert on evidence-based medicine. Professor of Epidemiology at the University of Sydney, he has published widely in international medical journals. He is frequently invited to review evidence for the development of clinical guidelines and to serve on committees developing health policies. Professor Irwig has developed programmes to teach medical students and medical practitioners how to assess research and make health decisions. For this work, he received an Excellence in Teaching Award at the University of Sydney. He has also run courses to help journalists and the public understand how to interpret and use health information.

Judy Irwig has devoted a large part of her career to writing and recording songs for children, conveying important messages about relationships, self-respect and respect for the environment. She brings to this partnership the perspective of a healthcare consumer. Her non-medical background allows her to explain ideas clearly without resorting to technical jargon or making assumptions that often come from years of professional training

Lyndal Trevena MB BS(HONS), PhD is a general practitioner and a Senior Lecturer in the School of Public Health at the University of Sydney. She is interested in making evidence-based practice more feasible for busy clinicians and their patients, and ensuring that good quality information is at hand for making decisions with individual patients. Information about her research and other publications can be found at www.medfac.usyd.edu.au/people/academics/profiles/lyndalt.php. Information about her practice can be found at www.gpcremorne.com.au. Decision aids and resources can be found at www.health.usyd.edu.au/shdg.

Melissa Sweet is an Australian writer and journalist, who has been reporting on health and medical issues for more than 15 years.

Before you read this book

We have designed this book to cover a range of health interests. It is easiest to read at the start and becomes more complex as it progresses. Depending on your needs and level of knowledge, you may choose the appropriate parts or chapters without necessarily reading from cover to cover.

Part I: Health advice can be harmful gives an introduction to the reasons why health advice may be misleading. It discusses some of the common pitfalls for consumers and health professionals, how to identify meaningful health claims and research, and why it can be unwise to rely on the opinions of the experts.

Part II: Your body, your choice is for you if you feel you have an understanding of the pitfalls in health advice, but need to know how to make better decisions by asking the right questions. It discusses the five key questions (see next page) to help make the best possible health decisions and what to look for when choosing a practitioner.

Parts III–VI are for you if you're satisfied with your decision-making skills but need help in assessing whether your sources of information are reliable.

Part III: Stories and studies introduces the concepts of what features combine to make a good study.

Part IV: Evaluating the evidence deals with which study designs best answer questions such as whether a treatment works or what causes a disease.

Part V: Improving your healthcare explains where and how to find reliable evidence and how to use it, and suggests ways in which consumers can get involved in improving their health and healthcare services.

Part VI: Testing your skill starts with an opportunity to practise your skills on a range of articles from the media, internet and papers in the medical literature. Later chapters are for you if you want a more advanced understanding of numerical concepts underlying health decisions.

There is a glossary at the end of the book.

There are five questions that we suggest you ask when making a smart health choice. They form the core of this book and are covered in detail in Chapter 5. They are:

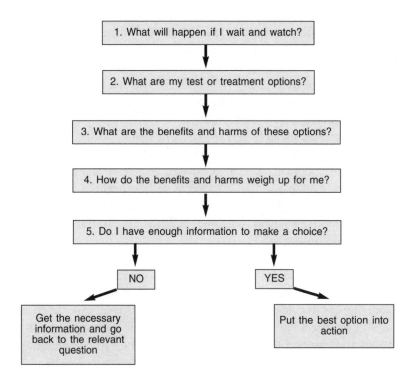

Acknowledgements

The idea for this book was conceived more than 15 years ago when Judy Irwig began to realise how fortunate she was to have an epidemiologist for a husband. When so many other people that she knew were floundering in a sea of often conflicting and confusing health information, Judy was able to ask Les to help her evaluate health advice. Often, Judy was surprised to discover that health information that was being widely circulated, whether in the media or by friends or even health professionals, was not reliable.

As Judy's skills in appraising health advice developed, she began to think that everyone should have access to the same sort of information that she did. And so she started work on the themes of this book. Judy and Les then invited Melissa Sweet, a journalist who had written widely about evidence-based healthcare and the importance of patients playing an active role in their health decisions, to contribute to the project. The result was *Smart Health Choices: How to make informed health decisions*, published in Australia in 1999 by Allen & Unwin.

When it came time to update the book for this more international edition, Dr Lyndal Trevena, a Sydney GP and academic at the University of Sydney, was the perfect person for the job. Her commitment to evidence-based practice and 20 years' experience as a GP gave her a powerful clinical and academic perspective on the issues so important for smart health choices. 'I try to communicate with my patients about evidence whenever I can,' says Lyndal.

This new edition contains many extra examples and sections. But Les is delighted that the core elements remain the same. 'This suggests that the principles we recommend as important for making smart health choices will be of enduring help,' he says.

The authors are delighted that the Australian cartoonist, Ron Tandberg's work also features in the second edition.

The authors would also like to thank the many people who have contributed to this book, directly and indirectly. For their thoughtful comments and their encouragement along the way we thank:

Joan Austoker, Hilda Bastian, Kathy Bell, Wayne Bell, Helen and Ray Berman, Maria-Ines Bruce, Sidney Buckland, Carol Chaitowitz, Iain Chalmers, Barbara and Jonathan Craig, Vikki Entwistle, Trish Greenhalgh, David Grieve, Sonia Irwig, Wendy Fine, Steven Fine, Paul and Nancy Glasziou, Kevin Irwig, Marcelle and Ken Israelstam, Sue Jackson, Andre Joffe, Danielle Joffe, Lyn March, Gill Muncke, Gerd Muncke, Andy Oxman, Sally Redman, David Sackett, Martin Stockler, Fiona Stanley, Martin Tattersall.

Les and Judy would particularly like to thank their wonderful family for their love and support, and for believing so wholeheartedly in this project.

Lyndal would like to thank Steve, Daniel, Emma, Ruth, Janice and Don for their endless love and support.

We also thank those authors and researchers from whose books and studies we have taken examples.

Disclaimer

The decision-making techniques and advice presented in this book represent the opinions of the authors based on their training and experience, and are not intended to replace appropriate consultation with health practitioners. Many of the examples and studies cited may be out of date by the time that you read the book. They are intended to illustrate various principles rather than to be used as a basis for health decisions.

The authors and publishers expressly disclaim any responsibility for any liability, loss or risk, personal or otherwise, that is incurred as a consequence, directly or indirectly, of the use or application of any comments in this book.

The characters in the hypothetical examples and the short story are purely fictitious.

I

Health advice can be harmful

1

This book could save your life

In the past, information was the real bottleneck, so any improvement in information would lead to an improvement in thinking and in the quality of decisions. Information access and handling (by computers) have widened that bottleneck. So we move on to the next bottleneck. This is 'thinking'. What do we do with the information?

Edward de Bono[1]

Every day we make decisions about our health – some big and some small, some conscious and some subconscious. *What* we eat, *how* we live and even *where* we live can affect our health. We make decisions about where to source information about maintaining good health, as well as about whom to see for treatment when we are ill.

We are bombarded with information about health on a daily basis. 'Good health' is highly valued and some people will go to great lengths to achieve it. Sometimes we worry whether we are making the right decisions and we seek assurances that we are receiving the best possible care. We often want answers to questions about a specific health condition. We might wonder about the meaning of certain test results, whether there are other treatment options and, if so, how effective they are. More and more people are also beginning to question whether tests and treatments might have side effects or involve risks.

Public confidence in traditional sources of health care has been understandably shaken in recent years by a number of high-profile hospital scandals and claims of negligence. In the UK, a major enquiry found three heart surgeons guilty of professional misconduct when 29 babies died between 1988 and 1995, more than double the rate in the rest of England.[2] An enquiry into 29 deaths in Campbelltown and Camden Hospitals in New South Wales in Australia also found mismanagement, poor communication and under-resourcing.

Despite the intense publicity that usually surrounds such cases of medical negligence, these account for a relatively small proportion of the problems with people's health care. A much broader problem arises from the care provided by well-meaning professionals in a system that is so fragmented and complicated that it is all too easy for things to go wrong. It is estimated that as many as 30,000 people die in the UK each year as a result of medical errors[3] and that tens of thousands of Australians die or are seriously injured as a result of their healthcare. Seventeen per cent of hospital admissions are associated with an adverse event caused by healthcare management.[4] In the USA, it has been estimated that about 180,000 people die each year partly as a result of their healthcare – the equivalent of three jumbo jet crashes every 2 days. These figures suggest that there is a great deal of room to improve the healthcare that many people receive.

Some people assume that complementary or 'natural' therapies provide a safer alternative to conventional options. However, there are many examples of people suffering side effects or complications from such therapies, whether from herbal products, acupuncture or chiropractic. In Australia in 2003 hundreds of vitamin and other products had to be recalled after 19 people were hospitalised and 87 reported feeling ill after taking a 'natural' travel sickness pill. Some alternative therapies can also interact with other medicines. Prince Charles sparked debate in May 2006 when he advocated greater access to complementary therapies at the World Health Assembly in Geneva and through the Smallwood report, which was commissioned by him. Some of Britain's leading doctors followed with a letter to NHS trusts urging them to fund only therapies that were based on scientific evidence. They were particularly concerned about NHS funds being used for homeopathic treatments, given that research has not shown them to be effective and patients were not being told this.[5] Early in 2007, a £200,000 pilot project of complementary therapies in Northern Ireland general practice had doctors complaining that the limited government health funds could be better spent on breast cancer drugs that have been shown to be effective in scientific studies.

This book will help you to evaluate the potential benefits and harms of various therapies, whether they are part of western medicine or a traditional or complementary practice. When making smart health choices, you should bear in mind what we *don't* know as well as what we *do* know about the pros and cons associated with use.

Although many cases of harm result from human and/or system errors, there are many other ways in which harm can be done. Sometimes, bad things simply happen by chance and are unavoidable. In other cases, they are caused by the well-meaning, but ill-informed, use of treatments and tests that do more harm than good. In addition to this, there are tens of thousands of people who, although not being harmed by their care, are not receiving the best possible treatment for their situation. Studies in many countries have shown that the way the same condition is treated can vary dramatically, depending on where the patient lives or on which type of doctor or health practitioner they see. Much remains unknown about how best to prevent or treat many common conditions; however, there is widespread evidence that the information that is already available is often not put to best use.[6]

This situation has come about for many reasons. Historically, the medical and health professions have not placed sufficient emphasis on the proper evaluation of health practices, although evidence-based practice has become much more common in recent times. Commercial interests, such as pharmaceutical and medical technology companies, often drive the introduction of new practices before their harms and benefits have been carefully investigated. (More about that through the rofecoxib arthritis drug story later.) The media often disseminate misleading and even dangerous health information. And consumers themselves often seek out and recommend the use of ineffective and even harmful remedies, perhaps encouraged by misleading advertising, websites or the advice of well-intentioned friends and family.

This book aims to help consumers and practitioners develop the skills to assess health advice – and hopefully to make decisions that will improve the quality of their care. For some people, making better-informed decisions could be life saving. We hope that it will be useful if you are struggling to come to terms with an illness or injury, and the best ways of managing it. Or you may simply want to lead a healthier life, and may be wondering how to make sense of the often conflicting flood of health information that deluges us every day, through the media, and from our friends and health practitioners.

Medicine has a long history of introducing new treatments and other interventions before they have been properly evaluated and proved beneficial. In the late 1950s, American surgeons began introducing a new treatment for people with stomach ulcers that involved freezing the stomach. The first few patients so treated showed a dramatic improvement in ulcer symptoms, and the technique was enthusiastically adopted and used on tens of thousands of ulcer patients. When a proper evaluation was finally conducted, it found that subsequent surgery for ulcers, bleeding from the stomach or hospitalisation for severe pain occurred in 51 per cent of the patients randomly allocated to stomach freezing – compared with 44 per cent of patients randomly allocated to a sham treatment (placebo). (The quality of research is increased by random allocation of patients – for example, by the flip of a coin – to either an active treatment or a placebo treatment, or a comparative treatment.) Needless to say, the stomach freezing procedure was rapidly abandoned, but only after tens of thousands of people with ulcers received the wrong treatment because of insufficient evidence.

Sometimes, the widespread introduction of unproven treatments has had disastrous consequences. In the 1980s, a new treatment for a heart disorder is estimated to have killed tens of thousands of people. This disaster, described by Thomas Moore in his book *Deadly Medicine*,[7] might have been prevented if the drug, flecainide, had been properly evaluated before its widespread use to control irregular heartbeats after a heart attack. It might have been prevented if more practitioners and consumers had been prepared to ask 'What is the evidence to support the use of this new drug?' The drug was approved for marketing after its manufacturer showed that it stopped several kinds of irregular heartbeats. However, it was introduced before studies had investigated whether this meant that it would also prevent deaths. When this research was finally done, it showed that the treatment had the opposite effect to that expected: it caused deaths.[8]

Unfortunately there are more recent examples of widely used treatments proving to be harmful after more rigorous evaluation has been conducted. Two examples that we will consider in more detail later in this book are the withdrawal of rofecoxib, an anti-inflammatory medicine used for arthritis, which was found to increase the risk of heart attacks and strokes, and the change in use of hormone replacement therapy after the results of a large randomised trial called the Women's Health Initiative (WHI).

This book is in no way intended as a do-it-yourself guide to becoming your own doctor. It is hoped, however, that it will help you to assess health advice better by showing you how to recognise useful evidence and reject that which is likely to be harmful. Its underlying argument – that we should remain cautious about any intervention that has not been thoroughly investigated and proved to do more good than harm – applies to all health advice, whether it comes from mainstream medicine or complementary/alternative practitioners.

The book is based on the philosophy that consumers have a right to develop a health partnership with their practitioner, so that all decisions take account of their personal preferences, as well as being based on accurate information about the beneficial and harmful effects of interventions. We hope that it will enlighten and empower those who may be feeling disgruntled with their healthcare, or who are confused by all the conflicting opinions and information that they are given, or who feel that their practitioners are not taking their viewpoints into account. The book will also be useful to readers making health decisions on their own, without consulting a practitioner.

We believe that the information in this book could have a profound impact on your health by offering simple tools to distin-

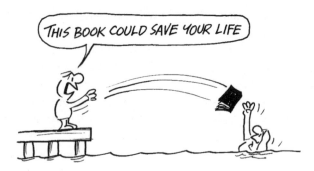

guish between good advice and potentially harmful advice. This knowledge could mean the difference between choosing the most effective treatment or choosing one that may be useless or even life threatening. Perhaps this book will save your life – or that of someone close to you.

References

1. de Bono E. *Parallel Thinking*. London: Penguin, 1994.
2. The Bristol Royal Infirmary Inquiry, 2001: www.bristol-inquiry.org.uk/
3. Weingart SN, Wilson RMcL, Gibberd RW, Harrison B. Epidemiology of medical error. *BMJ* 2000;**320**: 774–777.
4. Wilson R, Runciman W, Gibberd R, Harrison B, Newby L, Hamilton J. The quality in Australian Health Care Study. *Med J Australia* 1995;**163**:458–71.
5. BBC News. Doctors attack 'bogus' therapies, 23 May 2006.
6. Antman M, Lau J, Kupelnick B, Mosteller F, Chalmers T. A comparison of results of meta-analyses of randomised trials and recommendations of clinical experts. *JAMA* 1992;**268**:240–8.
7. Moore T. D*eadly Medicine: Why tens of thousands of patients died in America's Worst drug disaster*. New York: Simon & Shuster, 1995.
8. CAST (Cardiac Arrhythmia Suppression Trial (CAST) Investigators). Preliminary report: Effect of encainide and flecainide on mortality in a randomized trial of arrhythmia suppression after myocardial infarction. *N Engl J Med* 1989;**321**:406–12.

2

Be sceptical

What has not been examined impartially has not been well examined. Scepticism is therefore the first step towards truth.

Denis Diderot, Pensées Philosophiques

This chapter forms the basis of making 'smart health choices' because it encourages you to ask questions about the health advice that you receive – whether it comes from a television advertisement, a friend or a health professional. It will give you some of the tools to be sceptical, a critical thinker who can sift the misleading advice from that which has a genuine basis.

First, it is important to understand how our own biases can influence us. It is human nature to be tempted to believe explanations because they sound plausible, or because they agree with a prior belief or fit in with our value systems. Similarly, it can be difficult to give up a long-standing belief, even if not supported by the available evidence.

An example of this comes from the history of the tomato, which originated from South America and became a popular food in Europe by the mid-1500s. However, North Americans did not cultivate it until the twentieth century. They believed it to be poisonous, because it belongs to the Nightshade family, which includes some poisonous plants. The fact that Europeans had been eating tomatoes safely for centuries did not change their view.[1]

There are many examples of people's health suffering because of practitioners' failure to change their thinking in response to new medical evidence. It has been estimated, for example, that tens of thousands of premature babies around the world died or suffered health problems that could have been prevented had doctors been quicker to act on research evidence showing the benefits of giving corticosteroid drugs to expectant mothers going into premature labour.

On the other hand, new tests and treatments can be adopted *too* quickly, sometimes as a result of commercial pressure and sometimes for political reasons.

It is important to be critical of your own decision-making processes. Are you choosing or avoiding a particular treatment simply because that is what you or your family have always done, without investigating its harms and benefits or whether it is your best option? Be aware that healthcare practitioners also have their own personal and professional biases; a chiropractor will take a different approach to back pain to a surgeon, whereas cardiologists may have different views from liver specialists about the health impact of alcohol.

But perhaps you should reserve your most sceptical thinking for what you read or hear in the media. Consider a news report that cites a professor saying that the latest research suggests that drug *x* is a breakthrough new treatment for high blood pressure. If the professor's views are being disseminated as part of a campaign by the drug's manufacturer, this is unlikely to be mentioned in the news story. Similarly, if you read a report where an expert is sounding the alarm about the safety of a certain drug, it may well be that the expert's views are being disseminated as part of a campaign funded by the manufacturer of an opposition drug. Again that will not necessarily be mentioned in the news story. Such stories often do not put the experts' claims into a broader context – for example, looking at how they compare with other research in the area. And they rarely look critically at what evidence might be available to support the experts' claims. Clearly, it would not be wise to take such stories at face value.

However, many consumers and even health professionals rely on the news media for information about health. The problem with this is that 'news', by its very definition, is that which is unusual, sensational, scandalous or stirring. The media's preoccupation with rare, sensational events tends to make us lose perspective of what is normal. News is also susceptible to distortion and misinterpretation. The media are more likely to report studies with a 'positive' finding, such as those linking power lines to childhood cancer. 'Negative' studies – those finding no link – are much less likely to be reported. It is unusual for the complexities of health information to be accurately or fully conveyed in the media.

The media may report a new 'breakthrough' study showing that one treatment increased the survival of people with cancer by 10 per cent. It may not mention, however, that what this actually meant was that, one year after treatment, 110 of 1000 patients were alive instead of the 100 of 1000 who would have survived without treatment. Furthermore, it may not mention that what this meant for longer-term survival was unclear, and that the usefulness of the treatment was still uncertain because of its side effects.

Media coverage of health-related news can have significant effects on people's health behaviour. After Kylie Minogue's diagnosis of breast cancer there was a 20-fold increase in average daily television time given to breast cancer over a 2-week period. Messages during this time emphasised that breast cancer can 'strike at any age'. Although to some extent this is true, this message fails to point out that, while breast cancer *does* occur in women under the age of 40, it is much less common than in older women. Accompanying media messages at this time were critical of the government for not extending free mammograms to women of all ages. However, they neglected to explain that mammography is not a very accurate test in the breasts of younger women who have not yet reached the menopause. They also neglected to mention that mammography, as with most tests, is not entirely without risks. After this publicity the number of women booking mammograms went up by 40 per cent. But the increase was much higher in women aged 40–49 years compared with older women aged 50–69 years (25 per cent increase).[2] In other words, the intense media focus on Kylie Minogue's breast cancer seems to have made some younger women overly anxious about their risk of the disease.

11

Most journalists and media managers are not qualified to assess scientific data and to discriminate between high-quality studies and the many studies that are of poor quality and dubious value. You can be more confident of the validity of a study if it is reported as being published in a well-known medical or scientific journal, but this is no guarantee. Reports of such single studies often fail to include the broader context, so that the results are reported as if conclusive fact, whereas they may be tentative and not in line with other valid studies.

And most journalists and media managers are looking for a 'story'; the stronger and more exciting they can make the findings sound, the more chance that their story will be displayed prominently. One journalist expresses it this way:

> Scientists who do poor studies or overstate their results deserve part of the blame. But bad science is no excuse for bad journalism. We tend to rely most on 'authorities' who are either most quotable or quickly available or both, and they often tend to be those who get most carried away with their sketchy and unconfirmed but 'exciting' data – or have big axes to grind, however lofty their motives. The cautious, unbiased scientist who says, 'Our results are inconclusive' or 'We don't have enough data yet to make any strong statement' or 'I don't know' tends to be omitted or buried someplace down in the story.
>
> *Victor Cohn*[3]

Advertisements also have a powerful impact on our healthcare, whether by influencing a doctor's decision about what drug to prescribe or by persuading you to buy a particular food or pill. Tips for avoiding the tricks and traps of advertising can also be useful for evaluating other forms of health advice.

And, of course, there's the internet! An ever-increasing amount of health information is now available to everyone online. More and more, people are turning to the internet to look up health information, to try to find out more about either their own health problem or the health of a family member, perhaps to double-check information that they've received from a health practitioner or to 'chat' with people who have the same health problem via discussion groups and 'blogs'. Health programs can be downloaded via podcasts and played through i-pods while walking the dog.

Below are some of the common strategies used in selling health messages, why they can lead you astray and how to evaluate them.

If it works on a rat, it will work on you

Many reports claim that a certain product has been scientifically proven to have various benefits. But the fine print reveals that the results come from laboratory or animal experiments. It cannot be assumed that these results will be relevant for humans. Different species respond differently to various treatments.

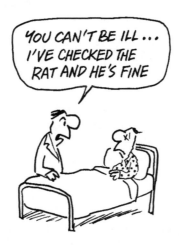

For years many scientists were convinced that taking supplements of the antioxidant, beta-carotene, related to vitamin A, would reduce the risk of certain cancers and heart disease. One of the reasons for their optimism was that animal studies had suggested that vitamin A was protective against cancer in some situations. The theory was strengthened by observational studies showing that people with higher blood levels of beta-carotene had lower rates of cancer and heart disease. But when proper trials were done –

randomly allocating individuals to beta-carotene or placebo supplements (dummy pills) – the results surprised many. An analysis of 47, well-conducted, randomised controlled trials showed that antioxidant supplements (beta-carotene, vitamins A, C and E, and selenium) do *not* reduce your chance of dying. In fact taking beta-carotene or vitamin A or E appeared to *increase* it.[4] To add further weight to this, another summary of the effect of beta-carotene on preventing cancers of the bowel, liver, stomach and pancreas also showed that it increased your chance of dying! It seems that, in humans, taking beta-carotene, vitamin A and vitamin E (alone or in combination) may do you more harm than good.[5–7]

Tip

You need to know the evidence proving that the product works on humans – and that its effect is relevant to your needs and situation.

Here's how it works

A remedy which is known to work, though nobody knows why, is preferable to a remedy which has the support of theory without the confirmation of practice. . . . The question to which we must always find an answer is not 'should it work?' but 'does it work?

Richard Asher[8]

People selling health messages, especially advertisers, love to tell you 'how their product works'. This strategy can be very convincing because it seems to make 'good sense' that, if we understand the mechanism by which something might work, the hoped-for outcome will automatically follow. But knowing how something is supposed to work is not proof that it does work.

For example, knowing that a substance changes the lining of your stomach, or plumps out your skin cells – these are examples of markers which are sometimes called *surrogate* or *intermediate measures* – may be intriguing, but is certainly no proof that you will have better digestion or smoother skin. These outcomes that matter to you are often called 'person-centred outcomes'. And on a more serious note, remember the story of flecainide, the drug that was meant to reduce deaths by treating irregular heart rhythms, but in fact increased the risk of death. What we really need to know is whether a product or treatment will improve our quality of life or help us to live longer.

Similarly, we should not discard treatments that have been proven to have benefits, simply because we do not understand how they work. Many thousands of women and their babies probably suffered unnecessarily because the medical profession was reluctant to accept that the anticonvulsant, magnesium sulphate, was an effective treatment for eclampsia because they did not see how it could possibly work. Eclampsia causes swollen feet, high blood pressure and fits in pregnant women, and accounts for about 10 per cent of all maternal deaths worldwide – about 50,000 deaths a year. A summary of the results of six randomised trials has shown that magnesium more than halves the risk of eclampsia and was better than other anticonvulsants, although there is a small increased risk of caesarean section (5 per cent).[9]

People who dismiss alternative health therapies because their mechanisms 'do not make sense' may be as misguided as those who believe a therapy will work because its mechanism suggests it ought to.

Tip

You need to know whether an intervention works in practice (empirical evidence). This can come only from seeing what actually happens to people who have the intervention. We get this information from good quality trials on people rather than from theory alone. Person-centred outcomes describe how an intervention affects your quality or length of life.

Blind you with science

Product promotions aimed at the general public and at doctors are notorious for using inconclusive or misleading research, wrapped up in scientific jargon, in an attempt to inspire support for a product.

And even if valid research is cited, you cannot assume that it will be quoted accurately or fairly. Consider this advertisement aimed at medical practitioners for a cholesterol-lowering drug called Zocor or simvastatin. In 1993 the pharmaceutical company brochure included this quote from a 1991 independent medical report:

> HMG-CoA reductase inhibitors such as simvastatin … are the most effective in lowering cholesterol levels and are more acceptable to patients than the bile acid resins. . . .

In its original form, what the report actually said was:

> HMG-CoA reductase inhibitors such as simvastatin *and pravastatin* are the most effective in lowering cholesterol levels and are more acceptable to patients than the bile acid resins *although their long-term safety and effectiveness in terms of morbidity and mortality have yet to be demonstrated.*[10]

Another example of how science can blind comes from an advertisement for Ponstan, a non-steroidal anti-inflammatory drug. The product was advertised to doctors in Pakistan as providing:

> … unsurpassed efficacy compared to acetaminophen [paracetamol] in fever control and better tolerance.

When challenged by the Medical Lobby for Appropriate Marketing (MaLAM),[11] the company agreed to withdraw its claim of better tolerance from future advertising. But it defended the claim of *unsurpassed efficacy* on the grounds that this meant it was equivalent, not superior, to other products – although most general readers might not understand it this way. MaLAM has been renamed 'Healthy Skepticism' and their website has some excellent examples of misleading advertising that you may wish to look at via www.healthyskepticism.org/adwatch.php

> **Tip**
> Just because it sounds scientific doesn't mean that it is valid. And don't assume that individuals or groups with vested interests will be objective.

Personal testimony and celebrity endorsement

Often an individual's experience is used to sell products. A leaflet for a homeopath's practice, for example, says that people such as the Royal Family, Mahatma Ghandi, Mother Theresa and Tina Turner visit homeopaths. So what if they do? Celebrities don't always get it right. Just because one person has had a good experience with a product or treatment does not mean that others can expect the same outcomes, or even that that person's recovery was a result of their use of the product. Anecdotal evidence can sound compelling, but is not a valid guide for decision-making, whether it comes from the experience of your next-door neighbour or a personal testimony published in an advertisement. Of course, such advertisements never publish the negative experiences with their product. What is needed is evidence from high-quality studies such as randomised controlled trials. For reasons that we discuss later, randomised controlled trials, in which people are allocated randomly to the treatment or an alternative treatment or placebo, are the most effective studies for evaluating the risks and benefits of health interventions.

> **Tip**
> As compelling as it may sound, anecdotal information can be unreliable as a basis for predicting an outcome. Ask to see evidence of randomised controlled trials.

Summary

- Just because a product works on rats, or cells in a laboratory test tube, does not mean that it will improve your health. The outcomes of a treatment or intervention should be relevant to people. They should tell you about quality and length of life rather than some biological measure that is supposed to predict well-being.

- Knowing how something is supposed to work is not necessarily proof that it does work in practice. We need evidence from high-quality studies on groups of people rather than from theory alone.

- Don't be blinded by 'science'. All too often what is marketed as 'scientifically proven' is based on questionable research. And be aware of the vested interests of information sources.

- What matters is not whether someone famous recommends a particular product, but whether there is evidence from randomised controlled trials showing that it is more likely to do good than harm.

References

1. Goodwin J, Goodwin J. The tomato effect – rejection of highly efficacious therapies. *JAMA* 1984;**251**:2387–90.
2. Chapman S, McLeod K, Wakefield M, Holding S. Impact of news of celebrity illness on breast cancer screening: Kylie Minogue's breast cancer diagnosis. *Med J Australia* 2005;**183**:247–50.
3. Cohn V. *News and Numbers*. Iowa: Iowa State University Press, 1989.

4. Bjelakovic G, Nikolova D, Gluud L, Simonetti R, Gluud C. Mortality in randomised trials of antioxidant supplements for primary and secondary prevention. *JAMA* 2007;**297**:842–57.

5. Hennekens C, Buring J, Manson J et al. Lack of effect of long-term supplementation with beta carotene on the incidence of malignant neoplasms and cardiovascular disease. *N Engl J Med* 1996;**334**:1145–9.

6. Omenn G, Goodman G, Thornquist M et al. Effects of a combination of beta carotene and vitamin A on lung cancer and cardiovascular disease. *N Engl J Med* 1996;**334**:1150–5.

7. Bjelakovic G, Nikolova D, Simonetti R, Gluud C. Antioxidant supplements for preventing gastrointestinal cancers. *Cochrane Database of Systematic Reviews*, 2006.

8. Asher R. Apriority. *The Lancet* 1961:12–6.

9. Duley L, Gulmezoglu A, Henderson-Smart D. Magnesium sulphate and other anticonvulsants for women with pre-eclampsia. *Cochrane Database of Systematic Reviews*, 2006.

10. Anon. Merck Sharp & Dohme's promotion of Zocor (simvastin). *MaLAM Australian News*, 1994.

11. Medical Lobby for Appropriate Marketing (MaLAM). Adelaide, Australia. 1996;**14**:7/8.

3

Bad evidence

I'm always certain about things that are a matter of opinion.

Charlie Brown[1]

Thinking straight about the world is a precious and difficult process that must be carefully nurtured.

Thomas Gilovich[2]

What would you think of a newspaper report that said that a certain substance caused many major diseases, on the evidence that 99.9 per cent of all people who die from cancer had eaten it and that most sick people had also eaten it? Would that make you a tad nervous about trying the substance? What if another article noted that 99 per cent of people involved in air and car crashes had eaten carrots within 60 days preceding the accident and that 93 per cent of criminals come from homes where carrots are served frequently? Would you stop eating carrots?

Although this (very much tongue-in-cheek) report might make you laugh, it raises a serious issue: health advice can easily mislead, even be harmful, if not tested by high-quality studies. Studies are not always designed so that they are capable of providing reliable information. And there are different types of studies capable of providing different types of information. This chapter aims to help you understand the basics of health research and to give you some tips for distinguishing between the different types of studies.

Basic research – testing ideas

Getting back to carrots, there are several different types of studies that could investigate the killer carrot hypothesis. So-called basic research is typically conducted in the laboratory, using experiments with cells, animals or human tissue to investigate underlying mechanisms of the body and how they are affected by disease or potential treatments. In the 1920s a laboratory-based study on dogs with diabetes laid the basis for treating humans with insulin. But the early cholesterol studies done on animals were not appropriate models because animals and humans metabolise cholesterol in very different ways.

Although studies in the laboratory can provide important information, it generally would be unwise to assume that the results are applicable to people until they are tested more widely in trials on people.

The media often carries reports of promising laboratory research – for example, of potential new cancer 'cures' – which provide less exciting news when they are eventually tested in randomised controlled trials. Not surprisingly, the hypothetical 'carrot report' notes that rats force fed with 20 pounds of carrots per day for 30 days developed bulging abdomens. Their appetites for wholesome food were destroyed. Perhaps this is another example of why we shouldn't be too quick to draw conclusions for humans from studies of rats.

Sometimes basic research is done on people to test whether a drug or procedure affects the way the body functions or reacts (for example, to test for a change in body chemistry or function such as the way muscles contract). Although done on people, this is still basic research because it is concerned with laboratory measurements rather than whether people develop diseases, feel better or live longer.

Applied research – does it work on people?

Studies involving people generally fall into three broad categories:

1. Observational studies
2. Intervention studies or trials
3. Summaries of all the best quality randomised trials.

Observational studies

Observational studies examine patterns of health and disease in different groups of people who are exposed to different environments or lifestyles.

Intervention studies (trials)

Intervention studies investigate the effects of treatments, procedures or other regimens, by intentionally changing some aspect of the status of the people in the study. These are *experimental studies* to see whether people who get the intervention are better off than those who do not.

The most reliable intervention studies are those that involve randomly allocating one group to an intervention – whether a drug, a new type of surgery or an exercise programme, for example – and comparing the results with those in a control group who are untreated or who receive a different intervention. These are *randomised controlled trials* (RCTs). Randomised controlled trials are often also called *randomised trials*. A trial that is randomised will always be 'controlled' because it will have a control group, but, be aware, a *controlled trial* is not necessarily randomised.

Interestingly, it was observational studies that helped raise hopes that one of the vitamins found in carrots, beta-carotene, might help prevent cancer, because it was observed that people with higher intakes of such vitamins had lower overall rates of certain cancers. But observational studies are not as reliable as randomised controlled trials; there is always the concern that there may be some other explanation. Could it be, for example, that people with high intakes of vitamins are more likely to be healthier anyway because they are also more likely to be eating other healthy foods and to be exercising and following healthy lifestyles?

Another example was the belief that hormone replacement therapy (HRT) would protect women who had gone through the menopause from heart attacks and strokes after the menopause. For years, many older women took HRT to help stave off these and other risks. It was observed that women who took HRT were less likely to have heart attacks and strokes. Just like the beta-carotene story, the opposite was found to be the case when a randomised trial was done. One of the reasons that results from observational studies should be treated with caution is the possibility of bias. Women who choose to take HRT may be wealthier, eat a better diet, exercise more regularly, smoke less, attend health check-ups more regularly, etc. Despite the best efforts of researchers to adjust statistically for some of these factors, it is impossible to account for everything and bias can creep in.[3-5]

The best way of dealing with this type of concern is by testing a theory using randomised controlled trials. Randomised controlled trials are the 'gold standard' for evaluating treatments and other interventions because the randomisation process – where research participants are randomly allocated (for example, by the flip of a coin) to either an active treatment or a placebo or comparative treatment – helps reduce the risk of other factors influencing the results. We can be even more confident in the results when both the researchers and the research participants have been 'blinded' or 'masked', so that they do not know who is taking the active treatment. Indeed, as mentioned earlier, when the randomised controlled trials of beta-carotene supplements were finally done, they suggested that, if anything, the supplements might increase the risk of some cancers[6] and the randomised trial of HRT showed that it increased the risk of heart attacks and strokes, particularly in the first 12 months.[4,5]

Randomised controlled trials also allow a comparison with what would have happened without the intervention. It is all very well to say that a new antibiotic, for example, cures 90 per cent of people suffering from a respiratory infection. But what if 90 per cent would have recovered anyway, without any treatment? Too often, however, we hear reports from the media and other sources that a clinical trial has shown such and such. What we need to know is whether this was a randomised controlled trial, because clinical trials do not always include a control group and are not necessarily randomised. The results of randomised controlled trials are available for many areas of healthcare and the number is increasing. However, if such evidence is lacking, you might have to rely on the next best source of evidence. Below are some of the other points that can help you evaluate health advice and, it is hoped, avoid common pitfalls.

Summaries of all of the best quality randomised trials

In 1971, a British doctor and epidemiologist by the name of Archie Cochrane wrote an important and controversial book entitled *Effectiveness and Efficiency: Random reflections on health services.*[7] This book suggested that many people were being over-treated in a well-meaning effort to do everything possible to 'cure' them. He argued that the systematic use of medical research, in particular, evidence from randomised controlled trials, should be encouraged, so that safe and effective therapies would be more likely to be used and ineffective and unsafe ones minimised.

Eventually he established the Cochrane Library which is now an online database and is available free of charge in several countries around the world, including Australia, Ireland, Norway, Finland and the UK. It is a database that contains summaries of the best research on treatments and covers a whole range of topics from 'acupuncture treatment for depression' to 'zinc for treating the common cold'.

These summaries are called systematic reviews. They are usually better than just looking at just one randomised trial because, if a number of trials come out in favour of a treatment, that means the theory has been tested and proved over and over again and the results are more reliable. Systematic reviews are also more dependable because experts putting them together usually disregard any randomised trials that have been poorly conducted and keep only the good quality studies in their summary.

An example of a systematic review from the Cochrane Library is one that summarises the results of 24 randomised trials (that involved 3392 people between them all) testing the effect of over-the-counter treatments for acute cough. It showed that there is not enough research evidence for or against cough mixtures and suggests that this should be borne in mind if people choose to use them.[8]

Common pitfalls to avoid when assessing research

Just because two events occur together, does not mean that one event causes the other

You may have heard about the guy who had a habit of clapping his hands loudly several times every few minutes. When his friend asked why, he explained that it kept the elephants away. 'But there are no elephants around here!' his friend exclaimed, dismayed. He replied: 'You see, it works.'

Because two events or characteristics are associated does not mean that they are related, let alone that one caused the other. Just because people with red hair and blue eyes are more likely to get skin cancer does not mean that their risk will be reduced if they wear coloured contact lenses and dye their hair. Red hair and blue eyes are associated with an increased risk of skin cancer because they are also associated with pale skin, but are not, in themselves, a risk factor for skin cancer.

Similarly, you often hear reports suggesting that one disease or another is the result of an infectious agent. For example, one recent study was reported as showing that heart disease may result from a virus because the virus was found in clogged artery walls. Is this convincing? Not necessarily. Even if the study showed that cells from diseased artery walls were far more likely to be infected with the virus, this does not prove cause and effect. It may simply be that the diseased cell walls are more prone to infection – in other words, that the disease may precede the virus.

As the benefits and harms of many modern interventions can take decades to become apparent, it is difficult for the general consumer and health practitioner to draw conclusions about the cause and effects of diseases and treatments without the knowledge gained from proper studies. If a young woman takes a 'morning after' pill to avoid an unwanted pregnancy, she may be relieved when her period arrives 2 weeks later. Her anecdotal experience probably convinces her that the pill has been effective. What she may not realise is that, even if she had not taken the pill, there was a 90 per cent chance that she would not become pregnant.

Even if two events are associated, the causal arrow does not always point in the direction that is intuitively assumed; the cause-and-effect sequence may be reversed. A TV show host overlooked this point when describing a study that claimed that families who eat together have better communications. The host assumed that, if dysfunctional families wanted to improve their relations, all they had to do was share meals. In fact, meal sharing may be an effect rather than a cause of good family dynamics – that families who get on well tend to share experiences, including mealtimes.

Anecdotal evidence can be unreliable. You cannot infer a general rule from a single experience – especially someone else's

Anecdotal evidence is often the most difficult advice to resist because it is based on someone else's personal experience, which can sound extremely convincing and compelling. If your next-door-neighbour recovered from cancer after a watermelon diet, that can sound very persuasive. But we already know the dangers of assuming cause and effect – just because she ate the watermelon before recovery does not mean that it caused her recovery. Remember, too, that only survivors speak: perhaps 50 other people died of cancer after trying the 'miracle watermelon cure'. Anecdotal reports can give an unbalanced perspective. Now, if there had been a randomised controlled trial showing that patients who ate watermelon survived twice as long that would have been a different story.

Some things get better on their own (spontaneous remission). It is impossible to know whether a treatment 'worked' unless you know for sure what would have happened in the absence of treatment

Say you take antispasmodics – medication to stop painful bowel spasms – for irritable bowel syndrome. If the symptoms disappear over a few months after the treatment, you might assume that the antispasmodics worked. But the condition might have improved anyway. Only randomised controlled trials will answer whether the treatment will help more people to recover than would have recovered anyway. In fact, a summary (systematic review) of 11 randomised trials comparing antispasmodics with 'fake pills' or placebos showed that there was a slight increase in the number of people who got pain relief: 46 people out of 100 will get pain relief with the placebo and 58 out of 100 will get pain relief from the antispasmodics. In other words 12 extra people in every 100 will be helped, but almost half of all people got better with a placebo.[9] On the other hand, six randomised controlled trials of antidepressant drugs for irritable bowel showed no difference between them and placebo.[9]

This example also reflects what statisticians refer to as regression to the mean. This is a tendency for values in nature to shift towards average – for example, children of exceptionally tall parents are likely to grow into shorter adults than their parents, closer to the average height. And children of very short parents are likely to become taller than their parents, closer to average height.

Similarly, an unusually high or low result from a medical test is likely to reflect a more average result on repeat testing. For example, if you have a very high cholesterol count on one occasion, it is likely to be lower at the next test, even if you do nothing about it.[10] To get a true measure, you should have several tests. This phenomenon also occurs because of the body's natural healing processes, which means that many abnormal states (of sickness) tend to shift towards the average (good health).

Put simply, some things just get better on their own.

Thousands of well-meaning John and Jane Does have boosted the fame of folk remedies and have signed sincere testimonials for patent medicines, crediting them instead of the body's recuperative powers for a return to well-being.

James Harvey Young[11]

The placebo effect is powerful. People often report an improvement on almost any therapy, even a placebo (an inactive intervention). This is why it is difficult to discern the real effects of active treatments without randomised controlled trials

In one experiment, patients with bleeding ulcers were divided into two groups. The first group was told that their treatment would dramatically ease their pain. The second group was told that their treatment was only experimental and little was known about its effect. Of the first group 75 per cent reported sufficient pain relief. Of the second group, only 25 per cent reported a similar benefit.

Both groups had been given the identical 'treatment' – a placebo containing no active pharmacological ingredient.[12]

What was at work was the power of the placebo – or perhaps, more correctly, the power of the mind. The placebo effect is a well-documented phenomenon, whereby the apparent outcome of treatment can be positively influenced by the mere expectation that it will work, held by the patient and/or doctor.

You might ask why it is so important to determine what produces the benefit. After all, does it really matter what makes someone feel better – the placebo effect or an active treatment? Of course, if placebos work that's great, but we want to know whether it is worth risking the side effects of any additional pharmacological effect of an active drug beyond its placebo effect.

Consider that earlier in the twentieth century many thousands of patients with angina (chest pain caused by constricted blood vessels) underwent various treatments that are now known to have no effect whatsoever. Many of these patients and their doctors reported remarkable (if not long-lasting) improvements after trying potentially dangerous drug treatments, and also after an invasive surgical procedure that involved tying off an artery in the chest.

This is one of the most important reasons for randomised controlled trials, which help discern the impact of the active component of a treatment over and above its placebo impact.

The placebo effect is generally seen as beneficial for patients, because it can improve symptoms. But it can also be responsible for harmful effects – what is sometimes called the *nocebo* effect. For example, some dentists say that controversy over the safety of amalgam fillings has had a nocebo effect. As they are worried that their fillings might be making them sick, some people have felt symptoms – regardless of whether their teeth are filled with amalgam or other substances.

Screening tests that detect disease early are not always beneficial. They can lead to people living more years with disease rather than longer lives

A screening test, as distinct from a diagnostic test, is used to identify disease in people who have no symptoms. This is great if early diagnosis of a disease will result in more effective treatment. However, in some cases, making an early diagnosis may not be helpful, particularly if there is no effective treatment. In many countries, the advent of tests to screen healthy men for markers associated with prostate disease has led to an explosion in the number of men diagnosed with the cancer. In the UK alone, the number of men diagnosed with prostate cancer almost doubled in the 5 years from 1990 and in Australia it tripled.[13, 14] But this dramatic increase is not believed to represent a 'real' increase in the cancer's incidence and is instead believed to reflect earlier diagnosis. Thus, there are more men who now know that they have prostate cancer, but not necessarily any more men with the cancer.

For some diseases, early detection does not help to prolong life because earlier treatment is no more effective than later treatment. In these situations, early detection simply increases the years of disease from the time of diagnosis rather than increasing years of life. This is called 'lead time bias'. To explain further, here is an example.

Andy is the same individual in all scenarios and this is what might happen to him in three different situations, as if they were happening in parallel universes (Figure 3.1):

1. Scenario 1: Andy decides against screening in 2000 and dies in 2010, 5 years after developing symptoms. He lives for 5 years with disease X.
2. Scenario 2: Andy is screened in 2000, found to have disease X and dies in 2010, 5 years after developing symptoms. Screening has not prolonged his life but merely increased the number of years lived with disease x from 5 years to 10 years.
3. Scenario 3: Andy is screened in 2000, found to have disease X and dies 15 years later in 2015. Screening has prolonged his life by 5 years.

From this example we can see that longer survival from time of diagnosis is not a reliable way of determining whether screening is effective. For this we need randomised controlled trials comparing death rates in screened and unscreened groups.

Dates: 2000	2005	2010	2015->
Andy is not screened	In 2005 Andy presents with symptoms and is diagnosed with disease X	In 2010 Andy dies having lived for **5 years** since diagnosis	

5 years lived
with disease X

| In 2000 Andy is screened and diagnosed with disease X | | In 2010 Andy dies having lived for **10 years** since diagnosis | |

10 years lived with disease X
Screening did not prolong his life

| In 2000 Andy is screened and diagnosed with disease X | | | In 2015 Andy dies having lived for **15 years** since diagnosis |

15 years lived with disease X
Screening prolonged his life by 5 years

Figure 3.1 Andy's three scenarios

Screening for prostate cancer is another good illustration of the potential for screening programmes to do more harm than good. In the UK and Australia, most authorities have not recommended that a formal screening programme be introduced for this reason, although there is a great deal of *de facto* screening occurring. (For further information about this subject, see the NHS Cancer Screening Programme's *Prostate Cancer Risk Management* website and also *The PSA Decision – what you need to know* video and booklet.[15, 16])

Here are some statistics that help explain why screening is not necessarily beneficial: suppose 10,000 men are screened by a PSA test, which measures the blood levels of prostate-specific antigen (Figure 3.2). Of these, 8500 will have a negative result, although 765 of this group can be expected to develop the cancer anyway, because the test is not 100 per cent accurate (and nor is any test).

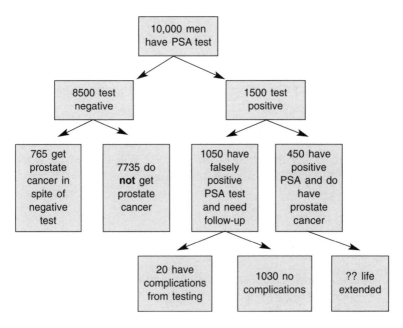

Figure 3.2 The consequences of screening for prostate cancer

Of the 1500 men with a positive result who undergo further testing, 1050 will then be given the all clear, although up to 20 may develop complications as a result of their further investigations and all could be expected to have suffered some degree of psychological stress.[17]

Of the 450 who are shown to have the cancer, it is not yet clear to what extent treatment will extend their lives or improve their quality of lives. Some will suffer serious consequences as a result of their treatment, such as incontinence and impotence. And because of the slow-growing nature of many prostate cancers – it is commonly said that most men die with prostate cancer rather than of it – it is quite possible that many men will have suffered adversely from investigation and treatment for a condition that may never have harmed them. The trouble is that we do not now have a good way of selecting which men might benefit from early detection and treatment.

The prostate cancer story is a powerful reminder of why you should always ask what the risks and benefits of any screening test are. Even mammography screening, which has proved to save lives when used to detect breast cancer in women aged over 40, involves some harms, and these may outweigh benefits at the younger end of that age range.

You should ask what is the chance that this screening test will accurately detect an important disease? What are the risks and benefits of earlier detection of the disease? Will it give you extra years of life, or just extra years of disease?

Summary

Assessing medical research can be complex – even for the experts. It helps to understand some of the more common pitfalls:

- Laboratory-based research on animals does not necessarily apply directly to humans.

- To test whether a treatment is effective in humans requires a randomised controlled trial on people who have the condition of interest.

- Just because health characteristics or events are associated – or occur together – does not mean that they are related, or that there is a cause-and-effect relationship.

- Anecdotal evidence can be dangerous. You cannot infer a general rule from a single experience – especially someone else's.

- Many diseases get better with or without treatment. It is impossible to know whether a treatment 'worked' unless you know for sure what would have happened in the absence of treatment.

continued

- The placebo is powerful. People often report an improvement on almost any therapy, even a placebo (a biologically inactive intervention). This makes it difficult to discern the real effects of active treatments without randomised controlled trials.

- Screening tests that detect early disease are not always beneficial. They can lead to people living more years with disease rather than leading longer lives. This is called 'lead-time bias'. (A screening test, as distinct from a diagnostic test, is used to identify disease in people who have no symptoms.)

References

1. Chalmers I. What do I want from health research and researchers when I am a patient? *BMJ* 1995;**310**:1315–18.
2. Gilovich T. *How We Know What Isn't So: The fallibility of human reason in everyday life*. New York: Free Press, 1991: 187.
3. Rossouw J, Anderson G, Prentice R et al. Risks and benefits of estrogen plus progestin in healthy postmenopausal women. *JAMA* 2002;**288**:321–33.
4. Wassertheil-Smoller S, Hendrix S et al. Effect of estrogen plus progestin on stroke in postmenopausal women. *JAMA* 2003;**289**:2673–84.
5. Manson J, Hsia J, KC J, Rossouw J et al. Estrogen plus progestin and the risk of coronary heart disease. *N Engl J Med* 2003;**349**:523–34.
6. Bjelakovic G, Nikolova D, Simonetti R, Gluud C. Antioxidant supplements for preventing gastrointestinal cancers. *Cochrane Database of Systematic Reviews*, 2006.
7. Cochrane A. *Effectiveness and Efficiency: Random reflections on health services*. Abingdon: Burgess & Son Ltd, 1971.

8. Schroeder K, Fahey T. Over-the-counter medications for acute cough in children and adults in ambulatory settings (Cochrane Review). *Cochrane Database of Systematic Reviews*, 2004(4).

9. Quartero A, Meineche-Schmidt V, Muris J, Rubin G, de Wit N. Bulking agents, antispasmodic and antidepressant medication for the treatment of irritable bowel syndrome. *Cochrane Database of Systematic Reviews*, 2006(2).

10. Irwig L, Glasziou P, Wilson A, Macaskill P. Estimating an individual's true cholesterol level and response to intervention. *JAMA* 1991;**266**:1678–85.

11. Young J. *Consumer Health – A Guide to Intelligent Decisions.* Times Mirror/Mosby, 1985.

12. Cousins N. *Anatomy of an Illness as Perceived by the Patient: Reflections on healing and regeneration.* New York: Norton, 1979.

13. Cancer Research UK. UK Prostate Cancer Incidence Statistics. http://www.info.cancerresearchuk.org/cancerstats/types/prostate/incidence/#trends

14. Sweet M. Fears of needless cancer tests. *The Sydney Morning Herald* 1996: Sect. 3.

15. NHS Cancer Screening Programme. *Prostate Cancer Risk.* http://www.cancerscreening.nhs.uk/prostate/index.html

16. The Foundation for Informed Medical Decision Making. *The PSA Decision – What YOU Need to Know.* Hanover, Hampshire: The Foundation for Informed Medical Decision Making.

17. Hirst G, Ward J, Del Mar C. Screening for prostate cancer: the case against. *Med J Australia* 1996;**164**:285–8.

4

Don't always rely on the experts

Medicine is indeed in the middle of an intellectual revolution. Methods of reasoning and problem solving that might have worked well in the past are not sufficient to handle today's problems.

David Eddy[1]

Recently a friend was describing some treatment that her father had been given. It didn't sound like he was doing well on the medication. When I suggested that there may be a more appropriate treatment, her response was, 'But surely a qualified doctor would know what's best.'

Unfortunately, it is not always safe or wise to make this assumption. It's virtually impossible for health professionals to keep completely up to date with the latest and best research treatments and tests. Gone are the days when a doctor could stay in touch by reading a few key journals each week.

To give you some idea of the extent of medical information overload, it has been estimated that about 560,000 new medical articles are published every year and 20,000 new randomised trials are registered. That's equivalent to 1500 new articles per day and 55 new trials.[2] There certainly has been an enormous change since the 1970s when Archie Cochrane and others suggested a more systematic approach to assessing health treatments through randomised trials.

Health professionals, like most of us, struggle with time pressures and face real challenges as they juggle clinical matters and the need to keep up-to-date with the latest good quality research. Even if they can access such information efficiently, there are many other challenges in communicating with patients about the pros and cons of various treatment options and finding out what the patient's preferences might be. This is not easy to achieve in a 10-minute consultation in addition to taking a thorough history and examining the patient!

This problem is reflected by the many studies that have shown a widespread variation in the rates of various medical procedures that cannot be explained away by intrinsic differences in the populations. Boston and New Haven, for example, have similar populations in terms of their healthcare needs. Most of their practitioners are associated with internationally renowned medical centres. Yet New Haven residents have been reported to be about twice as likely to undergo a bypass operation for heart disease as their counterparts in Boston, who are more likely to be treated by other means. On the other hand, Bostonians are much more likely to have their hips and knees replaced by a surgical prosthesis than are New Havenites, whose physicians tend to prescribe medical treatments for these conditions. Bostonians are more than twice as likely to have arteries in their necks unblocked as a way of preventing strokes whereas

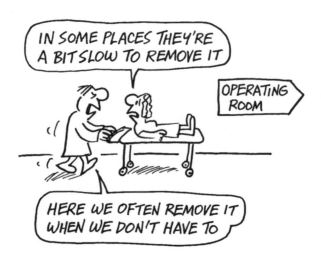

clinicians in New Haven prefer to recommend aspirin and other drug treatments. By contrast, hysterectomies for non-cancerous conditions of the uterus are more often performed in New Haven.

Other studies, in the USA, the UK and Australia, have found similar variations in medical procedures, which reflect different approaches to managing the same conditions. This may come about for a number of reasons, including differences in access to equipment or facilities, in training or in financing arrangements. But such variations can also arise because experts specialising in the same problems have different views about the best way to treat them. It is possible that some of those treatments are better than others.

But even if the experts did all agree about the best way to manage a particular condition, this does not necessarily mean that they are all correct – they may all be wrong. There are also dangers in relying on a consensus of experts – which has traditionally been the basis of many medical recommendations. Consensus may merely represent a middle ground between opposing views and may not accurately represent any expert view, or it may represent the views of the most persuasive or influential expert who might also be the most uninformed about the valid evidence. So we can't rely on advice or opinions just because they come from a so-called expert or 'a leading authority in the field'.

Why the experts disagree

It can be very confusing when the experts disagree about our healthcare. Such disagreement reflects both the complexity of healthcare and the uncertainty about what will be the outcome of a particular intervention.

Healthcare decisions are complex

When our grandparents and great-grandparents were raising families, practitioners had relatively limited tools and knowledge. Their advice was far simpler than it is these days, and the outcomes of treatment tended to be more obvious and immediate. Premature death was far more common.

Say, for example, your great-grandfather complained to his doctor of a pain in the stomach. It may have been caused by a minor gastric inflammation, in which case he would have recovered spontaneously within a few days, irrespective of treatment. Or it may have been a stomach cancer that inevitably would have killed him. In the first instance, the practitioner would have been praised for the old man's recovery and the treatment hailed as a cure. In the latter situation, you and your grieving relatives probably would have taken the philosophical view that some things are beyond the ken of doctors.

If your great-grandfather had been seeking help now, he and his practitioner would have far more information to consider and weigh up, including choosing from a wide range of diagnostic tests and treatments. Healthcare has become so much more complex, increasing the choices for treatment, but also increasing the chances that practitioners will disagree about which is the best option.

Health outcomes are uncertain

Another important reason for differences in expert opinion is the uncertainty of health outcomes – the same disease will have a different effect on different people. Nor can it always be accurately predicted how an intervention – whether surgery or a medication – will affect different people. Clearly, then, different practitioners will have different experiences. The best way of dealing with this uncertainty is to turn to studies of groups of people to find out what is the most likely outcome. This probabilistic evidence predicts the chance that a particular outcome will occur for a particular intervention in a given situation.

The complexity and uncertainty of healthcare help to explain why experts today face a new era: one that demands a high level of skill in evaluating information so that they can make sense of the growing body of research literature and apply the best available evidence to their patients' care:

> For centuries, the practice of medicine has been based on one huge assumption. The assumption is that physicians instinctively know the right thing to do. We call it 'clinical judgement' or the 'art of

medicine'. Somehow, the assumption goes, physicians are able to assimilate all they have learned from their medical education, their training, research, their personal experiences, and conversations with their colleagues, as well as all the information about their patients – their signs, symptoms, hopes, and fears – to determine the right thing to do.

David Eddy[3]

Fortunately, there is now an international push to ensure that health care is based on evidence rather than experts' opinions or consensus. Clearly, good healthcare requires that practitioners use clinical judgement together with the best evidence. Alone, neither is enough.

Practitioners may be poorly informed

Evidence-based healthcare is becoming more widely used by responsible practitioners worldwide. This has been possible largely because of the growth and availability of electronically accessible information offering practitioners and consumers previously unimaginable possibilities for making the best health decisions. The problem is that not all of this information is reliable. Much of it is based on poor quality studies. However, practitioners are being trained to access and assess the best quality of research.

Not all practitioners practise evidence-based health care

Although usually well intentioned, practitioners may not offer optimal care because many are not integrating the best available evidence into their decisions. This evidence is accessible through electronic databases, from good quality journals and from evidence-based guidelines.

Even when good quality evidence is available, not all practitioners are using it. This is partly because there are often delays between the results of research and the publication of easily accessible recommendations based on the research, and partly because old habits die hard. Many practitioners are resistant to changing practices that have become routine even when they may no longer be appropriate.

Not all practitioners know where to find the evidence

Practitioners might not know where to find the relevant, evidence-based information. Traditionally, many have relied on sources such as medical education, their own experience, previous and continuing medical education, and pharmaceutical companies – sources that are often inappropriate, biased or out of date. Indeed, medical schools have traditionally concentrated on the basic sciences – such as anatomy, physiology and biochemistry – and have begun teaching skills in critical appraisal of studies only over the past decade. There is an ever-increasing number of clinical practice guidelines based on the best available research but sometimes these can be difficult to find and to use with the patient there on the spot.

We can tell that many practitioners lack the skills to judge studies because of the fact that much poor quality research is still being cited as the basis for a large number of health practices and products. We should also remember that medicine has a long history of not recognising the harms of some interventions.

The most famous example is thalidomide – a drug that was considered to be safe enough to be widely used to treat morning sickness in the early 1960s before it was found to cause limb deformities in the developing fetus. But there are many more such examples – tonsillectomies were once commonly performed on children in the belief that they prevented repeated bouts of throat infections. A number of surgical deaths forced a reassessment of this procedure and a significant reduction in its use. Early in the twentieth century, babies' mouths were routinely cleaned in the belief that it reduced germs. Only later was it recognised that this cleaning caused ulcers of the palate. In the 1950s many patients with dangerously high blood pressure underwent traumatic surgery to remove the nerves running down either side of their spines. The operation was of doubtful value, but could cause terrible side effects. More recently, the antiarthritis pill rofecoxib was taken off the market when serious side effects emerged after the drug's widespread introduction.

'Safe' does not mean 'risk free'

So when a practitioner tells you that a treatment or test is generally safe, be aware that there may be harms that have not yet been discovered. 'Safe' often means that there are no known harms. And don't assume that, because something is said to be 'natural', it is risk free. 'Natural' and 'harmless' are not the same. Vitamin supplements taken in excess and some herbal products can have dangerous side effects, ranging from headaches to liver damage. As for any intervention, their harms might not be immediately obvious and, indeed, may emerge only after years of use or after large, high-quality studies have been done. As with any other intervention, their use should be handled with care.

Evidence can sometimes be distorted by drug companies

The story of the anti-arthritis drug, rofecoxib, illustrates a number of these points very nicely.

One of the difficulties facing people with arthritis is the fact that some of the commonly used anti-inflammatory drugs can cause nausea, belching and, even more seriously, ulcers in the upper

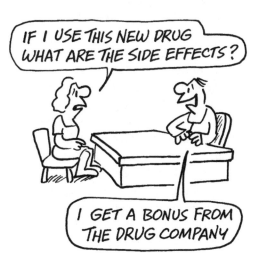

IF I USE THIS NEW DRUG WHAT ARE THE SIDE EFFECTS?

I GET A BONUS FROM THE DRUG COMPANY

gastric tract. A drug that would have the same pain-relieving effects but fewer side effects would obviously be desirable, and there was much interest in a newer generation of anti-inflammatories called the COX-2 (cyclo-oxygenase 2) inhibitors.

In 2000, the *New England Journal of Medicine*, one of the medical world's most prestigious journals, published the results of a randomised controlled trial (the VIGOR study), which included 8076 patients with rheumatoid arthritis. Participants were randomly assigned to receive either the new COX-2 inhibitor,[4] rofecoxib, or the more commonly used drug naproxen. That sounds good, you might say, having read the earlier chapters of this book.

In that paper, the authors commented that the naproxen recipients had a lower rate of heart attacks (1 per 1000) over a 9-month follow-up compared with the rofecoxib group (4 per 1000). Note that the other way you could report this is that the rofecoxib group had a higher rate of heart attacks than the naproxen group. This is called a framing effect. In other words, how information is presented or framed can affect how it is interpreted.

It was thought at that time, that the difference in cardiovascular event rates was caused by the fact that a lot of the heart attack sufferers should have been taking aspirin. They also claimed that naproxen itself was protective against heart attacks, a point that had not really been proved and was questioned by outside scientists at the time. The drug company that was funding the trial, the manufacturer of rofecoxib, contacted researchers who were conducting other studies with their drug to suggest that patients could use low-dose aspirin with it for cardioprotection if required. The Federal Drug Agency (FDA), in February 2002, added a warning label to rofecoxib packaging that it may increase your risk of heart attacks and strokes, but the drug was still available to the public.

As this possible link between rofecoxib and an increased risk of heart attacks and strokes became apparent in 2000, another study was getting under way to look at whether this same drug could help to prevent bowel polyps and cancers.[5] The researchers in that trial, which was funded by the same drug company (the APPROVE study), found that rofecoxib *was* associated with an increase in cardiovascular risk. Researchers took the preliminary results to the drug company in September 2004, the trial was stopped and the drug was withdrawn from the market immediately. Meanwhile, the drug company had benefited from a $US2.5billion revenue from rofecoxib sales in the year before the withdrawal. The FDA estimates that the drug caused between 88,000 and 139,000 heart attacks, 30–40 per cent of which were probably fatal, in the 5 years during which the drug was on the market. There have been over 100,000 cases and 190 class actions lodged against the drug company concerned and millions of dollars have already been awarded to plaintiffs.

Here is where the story becomes even more interesting and rather murky. On 29 December 2005, the editors of the *New England Journal of Medicine* published an editorial claiming that data about three extra heart attack cases had been withheld from the 2000 *New England Journal of Medicine* article.[6] The editors had become aware of these extra data when the FDA hearing occurred in February 2001, but had assumed that these heart attacks had occurred after the paper had been published in their journal and that the information was accurate when it had gone to press. However, after a drug company memorandum was subpoenaed for a court case in late 2005, it emerged that at least two of the authors knew about these extra cases well before the article was published and should have adjusted the conclusions. All three of these heart attack sufferers were people who did *not* need aspirin, thereby dispelling the original claim that. if rofecoxib were taken with low-dose aspirin in those who needed cardioprotection, all would be well.

Sadly, this is not the end of the story about misrepresentation of results from drug company-funded trials on rofecoxib. Not only do the claims of the VIGOR paper appear to be misleading, but there have also been doubts raised and a subsequent correction of the APPROVE trial results.[7] The APPROVE study had randomised 2586 people with a history of bowel polyps to receive rofecoxib or placebo. The trial stopped after 18 months when it appeared that the drug caused a doubling in the risk of heart attacks and strokes. As the drug company defended themselves against claims of wrongful death, they maintained that there was no increased risk until after 18 months of using the drug. In July 2006, the *New England Journal of Medicine* published a correction to its paper over 12 months after it had been published in March 2005.[7] In this latest controversy it emerged that people who dropped out of the VIGOR study early were not included in the original analysis. By omitting them, they underestimated the number of people who had earlier heart attacks while taking rofecoxib. The corrected analysis shows that the risk may increase as early as 4 months, and definitely long before the previously claimed 18 months.

At the time of revising this book, the rofecoxib story was still unfolding and we can only hope that many salutary lessons can be learned by journal editors, doctors and their patients about the pitfalls of relying upon trials that have been funded by drug companies.

Practitioners may not take account of their patients' preferences

> Over the last few decades, there has developed an appreciation that many interventions have significant harms; not all people weigh benefits and harms in the same way, and in the end it is the patient's preferences that count, not the physician's.
>
> *David Eddy*[8]

Consumers should expect that everyone who offers health advice or who delivers health care should provide sound information about the benefits of the intervention – whether a tablet, surgery or dietary changes – and the harms. Then you will be in a position to decide, with your practitioner's help, how these benefits and harms weigh up for you.

Practitioners do not always take their patients' preferences into account. This is often easier said than done and in some circumstances not practical or appropriate. It is often difficult to find out patient preferences in an emergency situation and, in some special circumstances, the law requires a doctor to overrule an individual's preferences if it puts him or her and/or others in danger. For example, an elderly person with poor eyesight and mild dementia may prefer to continue driving a car, but for obvious safety reasons this needs to be overruled. In most cases, a patient's preferences can and should be included in healthcare decisions. Later in this book we consider some tools that are available to help people become much more involved in healthcare decisions and help them to weigh up the benefits and harms of healthcare options. The fact is that not all people weigh benefits and harms in the same way. One person might consider a risk to be minor, although someone else might judge it unacceptable. As you become more informed about the evidence for different treatments and tests you may want your own preferences to be taken into account when weighing up the risks and benefits of a particular intervention. You should feel confident that your practitioner is considering YOUR preferences in decision-making, rather than other factors, such as what they have traditionally done in such a situation. The best way of finding the most appropriate balance between risks and benefits of health care is by choosing a practitioner who uses an evidence-based approach to health care and whom you feel comfortable questioning when making health decisions.

You should feel comfortable enough with your practitioner to ask whether any randomised controlled trials or systematic reviews of the best randomised trials have been done on a particular therapy. Remember, these are studies that are best able to evaluate the risks and benefits of an intervention because people in the study are randomly allocated to the treatment, an alternative treatment or placebo. Practitioners should try to run their practices so that they have sufficient time to attend to patients' questions, and there is no reason for competent practitioners to feel irritated or intimidated by reasonable questions from patients; on the contrary, they should encourage them. It may mean that they look something up for you if they have time during the consultation or, if they have a full waiting room beckoning their attention, they may get back to you at a later stage.

Given what you have read so far, about the rapid pace of expanding medical knowledge, you should feel reassured rather than perturbed if your health practitioner looks something up for you. They may even ask you to do some reading yourself and perhaps point you towards some evidence-based resources for patients. As patients quite rightly want to become more involved in their health-care decisions, the role of the practitioner will change and this is already starting to happen.

If any practitioner is too busy to answer your questions clearly or fails to help you find the evidence that you want, perhaps he or she is not the one to consult. And remember, 'practitioner' refers to anyone delivering any form of healthcare, whether a specialist, homeopath, dentist, nurse or counsellor.

Summary

Health and medical experts don't always get it right.
- They vary in their opinions and approaches to managing the same conditions. Their ability to assess and interpret health information may not have kept pace with the rapidly expanding amount of such information.
- Their views may be based on unreliable sources – pharmaceutical companies, the opinions of other experts, media reports and their own personal experience – rather than the results of good quality studies.
- It is your right that your health care is based on:
  – your practitioner's clinical skills
  – the best evidence from the research literature
  – your preferences based on the benefits and harms.

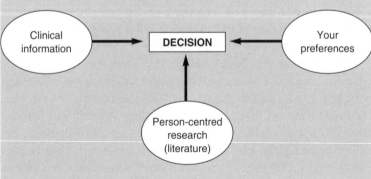

Figure 4.1 Evidence-based decision-making.

References

1. Eddy D. Medicine, money and mathematics. *Am Coll Surg Bull* 1992;**77**:48.
2. Glasziou P, Haynes B. The paths from research to improved health outcomes. *ACP J Club* 2005;**142**(2):A-8–10.
3. Eddy D. Medicine, money and mathematics. *Am Coll Surg Bull* 1992;**77**:36.
4. Bombardier C, Laine L, Reicin A et al. Comparison of upper gastrointestinal toxicity of rofecoxib and naproxen in patients with rheumatoid arthritis. *N Engl J Med* 2000;**343**:1520–8.
5. Bresalier R, Sandler R, Quan H et al. Cardiovascular events associated with rofecoxib in a colorectal adenoma chemoprevention trial. *N Engl J Med* 2005;**352**:1092–102.
6. Curfman G, Morrissey S, Drazen J. Expression of concern: Bombardier et al. 'Comparison of upper gastrointestinal toxicity of rofecoxib and naproxen in patients with rheumatoid arthritis. *N Engl J Med* 2000;**343**:1520–8.' *N Engl J Med* 2005;**353**:2813–14.
7. Correction. Correction to Bresalier et al. 'Cardiovascular events associated with rofecoxib in a colorectal adenoma chemoprevention trial. *N Engl J Med* 2005;**352**:1092–102.' *N Engl J Med* 2006;**355**.
8. Eddy D. *Assessing Health Practices and Designing Practice Policies*. American College of Physicians, 1992.

II

Your body, your choice

5

Smart health choice essentials

If you remember only the five questions discussed in this chapter when you finish this book, its purpose will have been fulfilled. Keep them in mind and refer back to them as you read the rest of the chapter. They form the basic toolkit that will help you put into practice many of the things that we suggest.

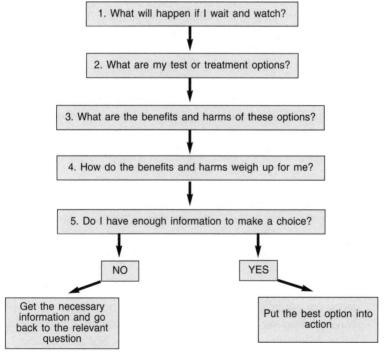

Figure 5.1 Five questions to ask when making a smart health choice.

1. What will happen if I wait and watch?

This explores:

- What can I expect to happen 'naturally' in my situation?

2. What are my test or treatment options?

This explores:

- What tests are available for people in my situation?
- What treatments are available for people in my situation?

3. What are the benefits and harms of these options?

This explores:

- How accurate are the tests in people like me? Could having the tests be harmful?
- How effective are the treatments in people like me? What aspects of my health could be improved by the treatment? Could the treatment be harmful?
- How likely are the benefits of treatment for me? How common are the harms?
- When could I expect to see these benefits and harms?
- How long lasting are the benefits and harms if they occur?

4. How do the benefits and harms weigh up for me?

This explores:

- What benefits are most important to me?
- Am I prepared to take the risks in order to achieve the benefits?

5. Do I have enough information to make a choice?

This examines:

- Does the available information answer my questions?
- Have I found out about all the test and treatment options that I want to consider? If not, where can I go to find out more?

Depending on the severity of your illness, and whether your practitioner has satisfied you that he or she practises evidence-based healthcare, you may not need to explore the quality of the evidence behind the answers to the first three questions. But if you do feel the need to validate the evidence to these questions, you will find the necessary techniques to do so in Part 4 of this book – Evaluating the evidence.

When we talk about 'tests' in this book we don't just mean blood tests and X-rays. In many ways, even having a health practitioner examine you is a type of 'test'. Similarly, when we talk about 'treatments' we refer to more than medication. 'Treatment' can include lifestyle choices such as exercising more or drinking less alcohol. It could also include physical treatments such as massage or heat packs or acupuncture,

We now take these questions one at a time to explore how they can help you make smarter health choices.

1. What will happen if I wait and watch?

A few years ago Lewis Thomas, an influential and thoughtful essayist on scientific matters, wrote that the dilemma of modern medicine, and the underlying central flaw in medical education, is the irresistible drive to do something.

Glennys Bell[1]

There is a natural temptation for consumers and health professionals alike to assume that, if something is broken, they should try to fix it. But many conditions are self-limiting – you will recover from them, and perhaps treatment will not speed up this process, or will only quicken it marginally with the chance of causing an adverse effect.

That said, good sense should always prevail. If the condition is likely to have serious consequences if no action is taken, it is probably not advisable to take the approach of 'watchful waiting'. Whether you decide to seek treatment may also depend on how much the condition is affecting you and your personal circumstances.

Bruce, for example, wakes up feeling rotten, with a sore throat and thick head. He recognises the symptoms of a cold, and considers his options:

1. He could battle on for a few days, going to work as usual, to see if it gets better without treatment. This option is called watchful waiting.
2. He could take a tablet to relieve his symptoms, knowing that this will not actually cure the cold but may make him feel well enough to continue his usual activities.
3. He could take a few days off work.
4. He could ask his practitioner for advice on other options.

As Bruce has an important conference looming, he decides on the fourth option to make sure that he does not have anything more serious than a cold and to get some additional advice on symptom relief.

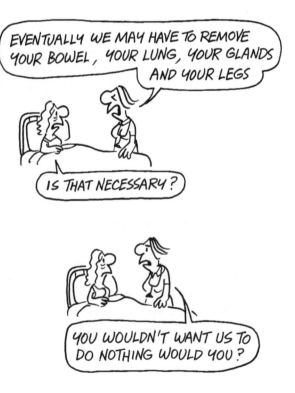

Taking this option may not make any more difference to Bruce's recovery than taking the first option, but his decision is affected by his circumstances. As watchful waiting is usually the first option, it should be the baseline against which all other options should be measured.

How you perceive the seriousness of a problem will determine how much time and energy you want to spend on the remaining questions: none for a trivial problem but much more for a major illness. Remember that the decision to wait and watch should be an informed choice, not an avoidance technique just because you cannot decide on another option.

2. What are my test or treatment options?

There are often many possible options for diagnosis and treatment, so it is a good idea to consider the most reasonable few options first.

What tests are available for people in my situation?

It is not always useful to have a diagnostic test – for example, if your condition is one of three possibilities, all of which have the same treatment, you may consider that it is not worth the time and effort to have tests. And the mere fact that a test exists does not mean that it is necessarily useful. For example, many people with acute low back pain are referred for X-rays, although the results of such tests do not provide a reliable guide to what treatment should entail or even to the cause of the problem.

Any test involves risks and most tests are not 100 per cent accurate. If there is a risky test for your illness but a relatively safe treatment, you might prefer trying the treatment first to see if the problem disappears. However, if there is real uncertainty about what your problem might be, and what is the best way to treat it, a diagnostic test might be valuable.

What treatments are available for people in my situation?

You need to know whether the treatments are aimed at curing the condition or simply relieving the symptoms. You may wish to consider a range of options from different types of practitioners, for example, your pharmacist, GP, specialist or homeopath.

3. What are the benefits and harms of these options?

Remember that you can only judge a test or treatment's benefits and harms by considering what would have happened without them. Finding out about the benefits and harms of the options involves asking:

- How accurate are the tests in people like me? Could having the tests be harmful?
- How effective are the treatments in people like me? What aspects of my health could be improved by the treatment? Could the treatment be harmful?
- How likely are the benefits of treatment for me? How common are the harms?
- When could I expect to see these benefits and harms?
- How long lasting are the benefits and harms if they occur?

It is important to keep these issues in mind for all options, whether considering a diagnostic test or a particular treatment.

How accurate are the tests in people like me? Could having the tests be harmful?

Diagnostic tests almost always involve some inaccuracy. As a result of this, a positive test result does not necessarily mean that you definitely *have* the disease, nor does a negative result mean that you definitely do *not* have the disease; there will always be some false-positive and some false-negative test results.

Say you decide to have a test for an infection. If the result is positive, you may have, for example, only a 60 per cent chance of having the infection – or a 90 per cent chance – depending on the test's accuracy. (In other words 40 per cent – or 10 per cent – will be false-positive results.) If the test is negative, however, you still have a chance of having the infection – perhaps somewhere between

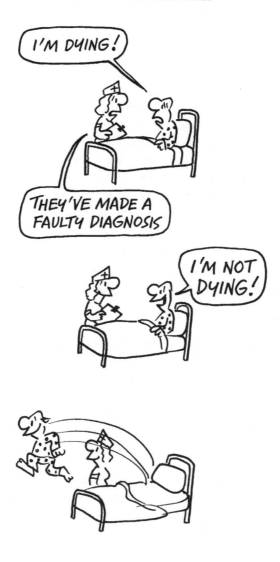

a 5 and a 15 per cent chance. This is why it is important to find out, in terms of *probabilities*, exactly what the test results might mean in your case. If your practitioner simply says the result means that you are at 'low risk' or 'high risk', you may understand these terms very differently from your practitioner, whereas it is much clearer if you are told you have a '10 per cent' or a '95 per cent' risk.

If your practitioner suggests that you have a test, you should consider asking these questions:

- What disease are you testing for?
- What do you think my chances are of having the disease?
- If the test result is positive, what is the chance that I do have the disease? Or, if the test result is negative, what is the chance that I have the disease anyway?
- How will the test result influence treatment of my condition? (If the result will have no effect on your treatment, you may want to think twice about having the test.)
- What are the potential harms of the test?

(For further information on the accuracy (sensitivity and specificity) of tests see Chapter 16. For further approaches to deciding when a test is worthwhile, see Chapter 17 on decision thresholds.)

How effective are the treatments in people like me? What aspects of my health could be improved by the treatment? Could having the treatment be harmful?

You need to know how the benefits and harms of any treatment might affect your quality of life and your survival, rather than what it is likely to do to your red blood cell count or your blood pressure – often called *surrogate* measures. Surrogate measures describe the results of different biological tests. They are not necessarily an accurate reflection of what is most important for you, the quality and length of your life – these are *person-centred* outcomes. It's important for you to know what aspects of your health could be improved by the treatment, not just what numbers might appear on a laboratory printout of test results.

Surrogate measures are used as markers for disease but do not describe the more important *person-centred* outcomes that affect how long and how comfortably you might live. For example, knowing that a treatment will lower your blood pressure, or that some diet will alter the bacteria in your bowel may be interesting, but tells you little about whether your pain will be reduced or your symptoms relieved. It also tells you nothing about whether you will live longer (on the benefit side) or whether you might feel lethargic, lose your hair or have diarrhoea (on the harm side).

Research has not, however, always examined the effects of treatments on person-centred outcomes; instead it often examines their impact on surrogate measures, such as blood counts. Sometimes, in the absence of evidence about whether your life will be happier or longer, you may have to make decisions based on the assumption that a beneficial effect on surrogate measures will translate into a beneficial effect on your health. For example, many people with HIV began taking drug cocktails because they had been shown to reduce the amount of virus in the body, but before it was known whether this would improve the length or quality of their lives. Understandably, as HIV is such a serious disease, many people were willing to take such medications because of evidence showing that they improved surrogate measures.

But such assumptions can be mistaken, as we describe in more detail later, with the drug that was widely used to treat arrhythmias – an abnormal heart rhythm that can occur after a heart attack. As people with arrhythmias are more likely to die after a heart attack than those without arrhythmia, it was assumed that giving a medication to suppress the arrhythmia would prevent deaths. When a randomised controlled trial was eventually completed, it showed that the antiarrhythmia drug suppressed arrhythmias but increased the number of people dying. Similarly, the drug mibefradil was taken off the market around the world after it became apparent that the drug, although effective at lowering blood pressure, could also cause serious problems when interacting with other drugs.

How likely are the benefits of treatment for me? How common are the harms?

You can never be certain about the outcome of any treatment; it is impossible to predict exactly what will happen to you when you have a disease or embark on treatment. What can be predicted, however, is *the probability* that a particular outcome will occur.

This issue is more complex than it might first seem. Consider, for example, the prediction that taking a certain drug will reduce your risk of dying from a heart attack by 20 per cent over the next 5 years. What if the drug is also known to increase the death rate from all other causes by 20 per cent over the same period? You may assume that this 20 per cent decrease in coronary deaths and 20 per cent increase in other types of death will balance out. In fact this may not be the case if fewer people die over this period from coronary heart disease than from all other causes combined.

Making an informed decision about whether to take this drug will depend on what is known about your risk of dying from a heart attack versus your risk of dying from other causes over the next 5 years. The probability that an individual will experience particular benefits or harms from the treatment is related to that person's level of risk. A healthy adolescent, for example, will have little risk of dying from a heart attack over the next 5 years so does not stand to benefit from taking a drug to reduce death from heart disease. For him or her, the 20 per cent increase in the risk of dying from other causes clearly outweighs the benefit of the intervention. In other words, a 20 per cent reduction in a relatively uncommon cause of death is not balanced out by a 20 per cent increase in a more probable cause of death.

At the other extreme is someone at very high risk of dying from a heart attack – such as someone who has already had a heart attack or who has unstable angina. For someone in this situation, the benefits of the treatment are likely to outweigh the harms.

Another example might be to consider by how much your risk of getting or dying from bowel cancer might be reduced by having a faecal occult blood test (FOBT) every 2 years. Several large randomised controlled trials have shown that doing this will reduce your chance of dying from bowel cancer by around 23 per cent. We also know that your risk of bowel cancer increases with age, and that it is more common in men and increases if you have a family history of bowel cancer. So if you are a 60-year-old man whose mother died of bowel cancer in her 70s, your risk of dying from bowel cancer over the next 10 years is about 13 in 1000 and this is reduced to 10 in 1000 with 2-yearly FOBT. If your risk is lower to start with, then the 23 per cent reduction won't be quite as much.

The number of lives saved by screening will be much less if you are younger and don't have a family history.

So it is important that you know not only the probability of benefits and harms from a particular intervention, but also how they relate to your situation.

When could I expect to see these benefits and harms?

Knowing when benefits and harms are likely to occur – whether they are likely to occur immediately or years down the track – can have a great bearing on their significance. For example, you may have to weigh up the immediate harms of chemotherapy for cancer – such as nausea, hair loss and discomfort – versus the chance that it will prevent future recurrence of disease and death.

How long lasting are the benefits and harms if they occur?

Knowing how long a benefit or harm is likely to last is important for evaluating its impact on your well-being. If a harm is temporary, you may consider it worth suffering in order to gain a long-term benefit. Alternatively, you may think twice if the trade-off for a short-lived benefit is a permanent harm.

An example of a temporary harm is a rash as a side effect of a treatment. When treatment stops, the rash clears. An example of a permanent harm is the loss of vision as a complication of surgery. This harm may not be reversible.

4. How do the benefits and harms weigh up for me?

> 'Would you tell me, please which way I ought to go from here?' said Alice. 'That depends a good deal on where you want to get to,' said the Cat.
>
> Lewis Carroll[2]

Many millions of people are willing to risk injury or even early death from jay walking. Yet many of these jay walkers would not

61

consider taking other risks with their lives that other people may consider to be minor.

How someone weighs up the harms and benefits of a treatment depends on many factors, including personality, history and circumstances. If you are desperate, you may be prepared to try a treatment that has a low chance of doing good, but a high chance of doing harm.

For example, a 50 year old woman may choose to take hormone replacement therapy (HRT) immediately to relieve menopausal hot flushes and night sweats. For her, the relief from symptoms that are seriously disrupting her life may outweigh the increased risk of 4 extra breast cancer cases per 1000 women if she takes HRT for the next 5 years.[3] Another woman may note that about half of women have relief from their hot flushes on placebo after 12 months anyway and be prepared to wait out the symptoms rather than chance the increased risk of breast cancer. We look at the research on HRT in more detail later in this book (see page 121).

What is important is that you have enough information to make an informed decision based on a sound knowledge of the potential for benefits and harms (quantitative information that your practitioner should be able to provide) and how important they are to you (subjective information that only you can provide). You also need to know how that compares with the potential outcomes of the other options that you might be considering.

5. Do I have enough information to make a choice?

If you are unable to make a clear decision, this may mean that you need to know more about the outcomes of your options or to consider other alternatives.

Does the available information answer my questions?

You could ask your practitioner if there are any evidence-based guidelines that cover your situation. (Evidence-based guidelines are based on a systematic examination of the best available evidence rather than on the opinions of experts, which, as we have seen, are not as reliable.) If an evidence-based guideline is not available, you could ask about the results of systematic reviews or randomised controlled trials. We discuss evidence-based guidelines briefly towards the end of this chapter and, along with the other study types, in much more detail in Chapter 10.

Many people also find it useful to speak to other people who have been in a similar situation, to get more information on their subjective experiences of the harms and benefits of a particular intervention. Remember, however, that different people experience things differently, so use their experiences only as a guide. In addition, such reports will not tell you how likely you are to experience a similar outcome. Your practitioner should be in the best situation to find out how likely you are to be helped or hurt by an intervention. If you are dissatisfied with the information provided by your practitioner, tell him or her that you still feel that you that have insufficient information and want some help with getting more.

Have I found out about all the test and treatment options that I want to consider? If not, where can I go to find out more?

You may need to think about other options if, for example, you have tried a treatment but had to stop it because you experienced a harm that was described as unlikely but none the less occurred, or if the benefit did not satisfy your needs. Or perhaps none of the options to date seems to have sufficient benefit for the harms.

If you need more information about your options, ask your practitioner, other practitioners or self-help groups. Many people find information from libraries, the internet and various electronic databases, but be aware that much information on the internet is unreliable. Later in the book we describe how to decide which information is reliable and list some good internet sites. Remember to compare new options with the best previous ones and to evaluate them with the same five important questions.

You may find it useful to seek a second opinion. There is no need to feel awkward about asking for this; most responsible practi-

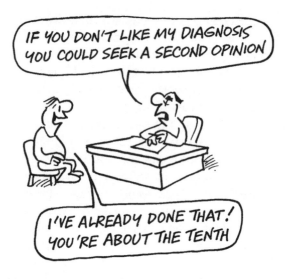

tioners will respect your right to see someone else. But be careful when selecting the number and type of practitioners whom you see; doctor shopping in order to get the answer that you are hoping for is not in your best interest. If you have difficulty making a choice, do not hesitate to discuss it with your practitioner. Remember, it's your body, it should be your choice.

An evidence-based guideline or systematic review could provide the answers to your questions

> Some doctors still believe, 'My practice is the universe'. But the idea that simply by observing our own practices we will know all the right things to do just doesn't hold water.
>
> *Jarrett Clinton*[4]

It is unrealistic for consumers to expect their practitioners to have all the correct answers at hand for every health problem. This is quite simply impossible given the complex and rapidly evolving state of knowledge. If it were possible, we could expect that there would be no disagreement among experts.

As long as health advice differs from expert to expert, some of it must be wrong. Practice guidelines have been developed in many areas to help address this situation. They guide the practitioner and patient on what to do in specific situations to achieve the best outcomes and avoid inappropriate practices.

However, many guidelines are based on a consensus of expert opinions rather than on a search for unbiased evidence. This approach is not reliable, no matter how valid the views appear or how eminent the experts involved. The advice of confident experts, which form such consensus guidelines, has a history of later proving to be misguided. Examples include performing X-rays on pregnant women to judge pelvic size, which was accepted as routine practice only a few decades ago. Today we would not use this test in such a potentially harmful situation when there is no good evidence of benefit.

The authors of evidence-based guidelines review the evidence from research and appraise its credibility in a way that most practitioners simply do not have the time or expertise to do. Ideally, practice guidelines should be set by a multidisciplinary group including health experts in the content area, researchers to assess the credibility of the evidence, and consumers to ensure a 'patient-friendly' perspective.[5]

We discuss systematic reviews further in Chapter 12, but for now will simply tell you that these are summaries of all the best quality randomised trials that have been done on a particular treatment.

Many practice guidelines are written with consumers in mind, so that they can be easily understood and interpreted by non-professionals as well as professionals. Summaries of good quality systematic reviews are also becoming increasingly available on the internet.

Examples of a consumer version of evidence-based guidelines are the information sheets on 'Evidence-based management of acute musculoskeletal pain'. The summary of research on treating acute low back pain tells you about treatments that have been shown to be effective, treatments for which the evidence is inconclusive or conflicting, treatments that can be harmful and treatments for which there have not been any studies.[6] Another example of a consumer version of evidence-based guidelines is contained within the PRODIGY *Clinical Knowledge Summaries for the NHS*.[7] An example of a website that summarises high quality systematic reviews of randomised trials is Informed Health Online (www.informedhealthonline.org).

What makes a guideline evidence-based?

Evidence-based guidelines should use the accumulated high-quality evidence from research on a particular topic and recommend ways to apply this evidence to individual people who vary in their preferences and in the features of their illness. Here are some 'ideal' criteria to help establish whether a guideline is of high quality. They have been adapted from some internationally recognised standards from the *Appraisal of Guidelines Research and Evaluation Collaboration* (AGREE).[8] *A Guideline:*

- should be recent, e.g. within the last 5 years. If it is not, ask if there is a more recent one. Guidelines may be updated more frequently depending on whether research has suggested changes in management.
- should be clear for whom the guidelines are intended and what they plan to address.
- should describe all the treatment options.
- should describe outcomes that are *person-centred* – about survival and quality of life.
- should describe both the benefits and the harms.
- should describe how the best evidence was selected and report the highest level of evidence for each recommendation. It may happen that a guideline's supporting evidence is not ideal because no strong evidence on the topic exists, but this does not mean that such a guideline should be dismissed out of hand. It may still represent the best available information. What is important is that a guideline's sources of evidence should be declared so that everyone knows its evidence level. The levels of evidence for evidence-based practice guidelines, from strongest to weakest, are:
  1) an evidence-based practice guideline or systematic review of all randomised controlled trials on the topic
  2) randomised controlled trials

3) other non-randomised studies on groups of people
4) case studies and opinions.

- Its development should have involved the main stakeholder groups across the relevant disciplines (for example, guidelines about managing a particular condition).
- It should be clear and accessible.
- It should be practical and relevant to its intended users.
- Its developers should have no conflicts of interest and it should be editorially independent of its funding body.

If all of these criteria are fulfilled, an evidence-based guideline should help you answer the five questions raised in this chapter.

Some people may still have some reservations about asking about the evidence behind medical advice for fear of implying a lack of trust. Many practitioners expect and welcome patients' involvement in their healthcare decisions and this is increasingly the case. Health decisions have become far too complex to expect practitioners to have the correct answer to every problem at hand. Increasingly practitioners are using evidence-based practice guidelines to care for their patients, so be confident in asking your practitioner about them.

Not only is it your right to ask about the evidence, it is also in your best interest to do so. Evidence is not a substitute for clinical judgement, but should be used in conjunction with it. Clinical judgement alone, without the benefit of evidence from high-quality research, is not always reliable – especially for important decisions.

The rest of this chapter explores a minor and a major health decision, to illustrate how the five questions might help you ensure (as far as possible) that you will be making the best health choice.

Applying the five questions: two scenarios

Scenario I: What should Fred do about his arthritis?

Fred, 60, is a retired engineer who is in fairly good shape apart from a nagging pain in his knee caused by osteoarthritis. Although there is no cure, there are many interventions that could help his condition: weight loss, exercise and physiotherapy, and pain-killers. As Fred is thin and fairly active, the most reasonable option in this situation seems to be the pain-killers.

Question 1: What happens if Fred decides to wait and watch?

Osteoarthritis may progress with age in some people. As with all health problems, watchful waiting avoids the harm of any treatment but also reduces the possibility of any benefit. Fred feels that the pain in his knee interferes with his daily activities, not to mention his great joy in bowling and playing with his grandchildren. He believes that the problem is worth treating unless the treatment side effects reduce his quality of life still more than the pain itself.

Question 2: What are Fred's test and treatment options?

Fred learns that non-steroidal anti-inflammatory drugs (NSAIDs) have long-term advantages if the joints are inflamed as in rheumatoid arthritis. But Fred's doctor has told him he was 95 per cent certain the diagnosis was osteoarthritis ('wear-and-tear' arthritis) without any inflammatory component. This was based on a physical examination and the history of an old cartilage injury for which Fred had surgery in his 20s. Therefore, the objective of treatment is to relieve symptoms and the most reasonable treatment option seems to be a course of pain-killers. The option of a further diagnostic test, such as an X-ray, seems unnecessary with such a high probability of it being osteoarthritis.

Question 3: What are the benefits and harms of Fred's options?

Like most of us, Fred has some previous experience of taking pain-killers for headaches and sprains. He knows that many are available over the counter and have minimal side effects. His pharmacist tells him that pain relief could be achieved with paracetamol and that NSAIDs, such as aspirin, ibuprofen, diclofenac or naproxen, are also often used for pain relief.

He then considers the benefits and harms of pain-killers – whether they will be long term or short term, how long lasting they might be and how likely they are to occur given his particular risk level?

Fred asks his doctor about the potential harms of NSAIDs and how they compare with those of paracetamol, which he learns can cause liver disease whereas NSAIDs can cause stomach bleeds and upsets. Fred is surprised that, although his doctor knows these side effects exist, he cannot provide any information on how likely they are to occur. The only justification that his doctor is able to offer for using NSAIDs is that many of his patients seem to be doing well on them. He tells Fred that, although several do complain of stomach pain, the pain in their joints seems well controlled by NSAIDs.

Question 4: How do the benefits and harms weigh up for Fred?

Making the correct choice is important to Fred. He knows that osteoarthritis is a chronic condition and that he is at the start of long-term treatment to control his symptoms. He is concerned about the possibility of stomach bleeds because he has had a stomach ulcer in the past. It is not yet clear to Fred how the benefits and harms weigh up for him.

Question 5: Does Fred have enough information to make a choice?

Fred is not satisfied with his doctor's suggestion of NSAIDs. When his doctor realises how determined Fred is to be better informed about the benefits and harms of the alternatives, he agrees to get some more information. A week later, Fred finds out from the doctor that there is a systematic review of 15 randomised controlled trials of paracetamol taken regularly compared with placebo and NSAIDs.

The trials show that pain decreased by 6 points more in people taking NSAIDs compared with paracetamol on a scale from 0 to 100. Paracetamol decreased pain by 4 points compared with placebo. There was a slightly higher chance of stomach side effects (nausea, heartburn, stomach pain) in people taking traditional NSAIDs (naproxen, ibuprofen) – 19 out of 100 compared with paracetamol 13 out of 100.[9]

Fred's doctor also pointed out that there is the option of paracetamol combined with other drugs such as codeine. However, these may be addictive, so Fred does not wish to use them.

On examining the results for his own situation, Fred is told that the risk of gastrointestinal bleeding is increased in people who have had stomach ulcers previously. As he had an ulcer 2 years previously, he feels that the risk is unacceptable for him, so he decides to try paracetamol to see if it controls his symptoms. If it does not, he may still need to consider NSAIDs despite their side effects because they are more effective pain-killers in people with moderate or severe pain from osteoarthritis. His doctor also finds from the Cochrane Database of Systematic Reviews that exercise can be helpful in reducing pain and glucosamine can have some benefits in the short term but by 2–3 months this is minimal. Both of these treatment options seem to have minimal or no risks associated with them so Fred will consider adding these to the paracetamol.

Talking to his friends about his decision to use the cheaper, safer drug, Fred is surprised at the number of his friends who are regularly taking NSAIDs without ever having evaluated their risks compared with the cheaper, safer treatment.

Scenario II: What should Pat do about her mammogram result?

Pat, 55, lives in a rural town and teaches physical education at a secondary school. She has been told that she has an abnormality on a screening mammogram that she had during a visit to her sister in another town. The initial positive mammogram was followed up by a recall for further mammograms, the results of which suggested cancer.

Let's see how Pat answers the five questions, with the help of the consumer guideline *A Guide for Women with Early Breast Cancer* by the National Breast Cancer Centre (NBCC)[10] and the doctor's version *Clinical Practice Guidelines: Management of Early Breast Cancer* (National Health and Medical Research Council or NHMRC).[11] These are the Australian guidelines that she chooses to use because the UK guidelines are not due to be published until 2009 by the National Institute for Health and Clinical Excellence (NICE). (The Scottish health department issued guidelines for clinicians only, in March 2007.)

The other excellent resource that Pat finds on the internet is an evidence-based decision aid from the Canadian Cancer Society called *Making Decisions about the Removal of My Breast Cancer* at *www.cancer.ca/ccs/internet/miniapp/0,3182,3543_16897665_19702640_langId-en,00.html*

Question 1: What will happen if Pat adopts a wait and watch approach to her abnormal mammograms?

Chapter 6 of the doctor's guideline compares surgery with doing nothing:

> Indirect evidence suggests that surgical intervention may extend survival from the time of clinical detection. In an historical comparison, women treated by radical mastectomy appeared to survive longer than women whose breast cancer was untreated.

The option of watchful waiting seems unreasonable for a life-threatening condition and Pat dismisses this option.

Question 2: What are Pat's test and treatment options?

Pat realises that a diagnostic test is appropriate for such a serious disease and she agrees to have a needle biopsy, which can be done without an anaesthetic and its attendant risks. The biopsy result confirms that she has cancer. A clinical examination does not find any lymph node involvement. Pat prefers to be treated near home so she consults a nearby surgeon who recommends a mastectomy (removal of the breast).

This suggestion comes as a shock to Pat who has heard that small cancers can be treated successfully by removal of only a portion of the breast in a lumpectomy, which is less disfiguring than a mastectomy.

She refers to the guideline for women, which says in Chapter 6 that surgery for early breast cancer involves either breast-conserving surgery or mastectomy and that, in both cases, lymph nodes in the armpit will be removed. However, breast-conserving surgery includes both surgical removal of the lump and postoperative radiotherapy to the remaining breast tissue.

Pat discusses her reading with her practitioner, who confirms that breast-conserving surgery plus radiotherapy is an acceptable option for Pat's situation.

Question 3: What are the benefits and harms of Pat's options?

The doctor's guidelines compare the two main surgical options in Chapter 4, saying that around 70 per cent of breast cancers are suitable for breast-conserving surgery. Pat has been advised that she fits within this category, so needs to consider both options. There is no difference in survival between women who have a mastectomy and those who have breast-conserving surgery followed by radiotherapy. Each form of treatment has its advantages. They say:

> About 1–2 per cent of women who have breast conserving surgery followed by radiotherapy find the cancer comes back in the same breast. In women with smaller tumours, the chances of the cancer coming back in the same breast are lower. Further surgery can usually be performed if the cancer does return. Some women who have mastectomy are happy to avoid the need for radiotherapy, and they may worry less about the cancer coming back, although they may feel more concerned about their lost breast.

Pat finds the interactive decision aid particularly helpful because it contains photographs of women after both types of surgery and provides probabilities for the risks of radiotherapy.

Question 4: How do the benefits and harms weigh up for Pat?

In Chapter 5 of the consumer guideline, it says:

> You are entitled to choose the treatment that best suits you. Before you make a decision, it's recommended that you discuss your treatment options with your doctor and any other people you may choose (such as family members or other health professionals).

Pat feels that it is important for her to keep her breast, for her self-image as well as for her work and social environment. But, for Pat, the personal cost of having radiotherapy includes more than the side-effects of the treatment alone. It will involve her travelling to a centre far from home for the course of treatment. As there is good evidence showing no difference in physical outcome between mastectomy and breast-conserving surgery plus radiotherapy for early breast cancer, Pat decides the personal cost of being treated away from the support of her family and friends in her home town is a small price to pay for keeping her breast.

Question 5: Does Pat have enough information to make a choice?

The guidelines provide contact details for women who want more information, or who may want to check the references from which the information in the guideline is drawn.

Pat is satisfied that she has had enough information to make her choice of conservative surgery plus radiotherapy.

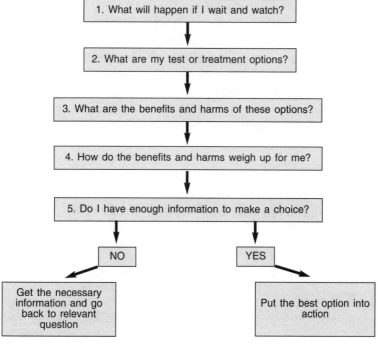

Figure 5.1 Five questions to ask when making a smart health choice.

Summary

Remember the five questions that will help you make an informed choice:

Question 1: What will happen if I wait and watch?

- What can I expect to happen 'naturally' in my situation?

Question 2: What are my test or treatment options?

- What tests are available for people in my situation?
- What treatments are available for people in my situation?

Question 3: What are the benefits and harms of these options?

- How accurate are the tests in people like me? Could having the tests be harmful?
- How effective are the treatments in people like me? What aspects of my health could be improved by the treatment? Could the treatment be harmful?
- How likely are the benefits of treatment for me? How common are the harms?
- When could I expect to see these benefits and harms?
- How long lasting are the benefits and harms if they occur?

Question 4: How do the benefits and harms weigh up for me?

- What benefits are most important to me?
- Am I prepared to take the risks in order to achieve the benefits?

Question 5: Do I have enough information to make a choice?

- Does the available information answer my questions?

continued

• Have I found out about all the test and treatment options that I want to consider? If not, where can I go to find out more?

References

1. Bell G. Doctors get better. *Sydney Morning Herald*, Good Weekend, 1994.
2. Carroll L. *Alice's Adventures in Wonderland*.
3. Rossouw J, Anderson G, Prentice R et al. Risks and benefits of estrogen plus progestin in healthy postmenopausal women. *JAMA* 2002;**288**:321–33.
4. Clinton J. Agency for health care policy and research. *JAMA* 1991;**266**(2057).
5. National Health and Medical Research Council. *A Guide to the Development, Evaluation and Implementation of Clinical Practice Guidelines*. Canberra, Australia: NHMRC, 1999.
6. National Health and Medical Research Council. *Information Sheet: Acute Low Back Pain*. Canberra, Australia: NHMRC, 2004: www.nhmrc.gov.au/publications/_files/cp94a.pdf
7. PRODIGY. *Prodigy Guidance on Acute Low Back Pain*.
8. AGREE. *Appraisal of Guidelines Research and Evaluation*: www.agreecollaboration.org.
9. Towheed T, Maxwell L, Judd M, Catton M, Hochberg M, Wells G. Acetaminophen for osteoarthritis. *Cochrane Database of Systematic Reviews*, 2006(Issue 1): Art. no.: CD004257. DOI: 10.1002/14651858.CD004257.pub2.
10. National Breast Cancer Centre. *A Guide for Women with Early Breast Cancer*. NBCC, 2003.
11. National Health and Medical Research Council. *Clinical Practice Guideline: Management of Early Breast Cancer*. Canberra, Australia: NHMRC, 2001.

6

Choosing a practitioner or a hospital

A few weeks after starting treatment for depression, Claire noticed a marked reduction in her libido. She was puzzled because the medication had helped improve her mood and enjoyment of life generally. She mentioned it at her next appointment and was surprised to hear that the antidepressant might be to blame. The psychiatrist explained that this particular drug affected libido in some people whereas other drugs appeared to be less likely to cause this side effect. On the basis of this information, Claire decided to try one of the other antidepressants. She wished her doctor had spent more time initially explaining the pros and cons of the various antidepressants, and resolved to ask more questions next time that she was in such a situation.

In this chapter we outline some of the aspects that you might consider in choosing from whom and where you will seek health-care treatment and advice. We recognise that different health systems will not always provide you with the type of practitioner or hospital that you would most want. This may be a result of differences in access for private fee-paying, as opposed to government-subsidised, places.

However, most health services are becoming more patient-focused and aim to give you a greater degree of choice. Although the National Health Service (NHS) requires British residents to register with a local GP, patients have the right to change doctors without giving a reason and many GPs operate within a group practice setting. Similarly, the NHS now has a policy that, when a GP refers a patient to a specialist or hospital for treatment, he or she can choose from several hospitals in the local area. In Australia, patients are free to seek medical advice including a second opinion without restriction, although choice of practitioner in some hospital settings is restricted if you are a non-insured patient. People usually choose their own pharmacist, dentist, homeopath and other health providers, but what is the basis on which we make these important choices in seeking health advice and treatment?

Many consumers are taking more active roles in their health care. The role of many practitioners is also changing, moving from one of professional paternalism to being a partner in their patients' decisions.

A survey of 652 Australian women in 2001 showed that 95 per cent of women wanted an active or shared role in treatment decisions about their healthcare.[1] Slightly lower figures were reported in a European survey, but still a majority of 74 per cent people preferred some active involvement in healthcare treatment decisions.[2]

In 2004, The UK Department of Health launched a program called *Better information, better choices, better health: putting information at the centre of health.*[3]

It is a three-year program underpinned by four principles. People should:

1. have access to accurate, high quality, comprehensive information delivered in the way they want
2. have their personal information needs considered and discussed at every contact with health professionals
3. receive as much support as they want to access and understand information

4. be empowered to ask questions and be involved as far as they want in making decision about, for example, the benefits and risks of action and how any risks can be mitigated.

The patient–practitioner partnership encourages and depends on a level of trust that demands mutual respect, clear concise communication and shared responsibility. Finding a practitioner with whom you can establish this partnership may take some time and effort, but ultimately it is in your best interests to make this choice carefully. You may have already found one, but may not have been taking full advantage of your role in the relationship. One of the aims of this book is to help you do that confidently. In other words, choosing a practitioner may include looking beyond technical expertise and also include considering decision-making expertise.

It is also important to consider your role in the broader community. When communicating one to one with your health professional about the best treatment options for your situation, it can be easy to forget that your decisions can have an impact on others. These may include your family and those who are close to you, as well as people in your workplace, school or wider community. There is often a conflict or tension between what may be your own personal preference and what may be best at a societal level – and there are no easy answers to this one.

For example, some parents choose to exercise their right not to immunise their children but this potentially puts very young babies and children with immune deficiencies at risk of disease. Similarly it is understandable that a patient with cancer might want the government to fund a new, expensive and not yet proven treatment in order to give them a chance of increased survival. However, when health budgets are limited this may divert funding from other health problems. This may lead to other people being indirectly penalised. These are difficult issues and not ones that can necessarily be resolved by individual patients but it is worth bearing them in mind. You may feel daunted by the idea of 'examining your doctor' in the way that we suggest in the following pages, but just ask whatever you are comfortable with. As time goes by and you ask about more issues, it will become easier.

Judging a practitioner's decision-making expertise

Competent decision-making expertise involves good clinical judgement to make a diagnosis and the proper use of evidence combined with patient preferences to choose the best course of action. However, not all practitioners approach decision-making this way. Although it is probably true to say that most practitioners can diagnose common illnesses fairly accurately, they vary in their ability to use evidence appropriately to decide what intervention – if any – is best and in their willingness to take account of patients' preferences.

Consider an elderly man who is considering whether to have surgery for an enlarged prostate. There is good evidence that an enlarged prostate is not life threatening, although it can be a nuisance. The potential side effects of surgery include impotence. A practitioner should be able to present information about the benefits and harms of surgery, but only you can decide which harm is the most acceptable – increased frequency and urgency of urination from an enlarged prostate or possible sexual dysfunction and incontinence from the surgery.

To help you judge whether your practitioner has good decision-making skills consider whether he or she:

* uses the best evidence available
* readily shares information with you
* takes adequate account of your preferences.

Does your practitioner use the best evidence available?

If your practitioner is using the best evidence available, he or she should be regularly updating his or her practice using the results of randomised controlled trials. Many practitioners say that they already practise evidence-based medicine, but, unless they make a conscious effort to keep abreast of the latest results from randomised controlled trials, you cannot be sure that their advice is really based on the best evidence.

There is no easy way of testing your practitioner's approach to evidence-based care without discussing it openly. You might start by asking their opinion on some treatment that you have found on the internet or been told about by friends. See if the practitioner evaluates it taking account of whether the effect of interventions has been tested in randomised controlled trials, and whether he or she talks about outcomes that matter, such as survival and quality of life. If practitioners do not update their practice from randomised controlled trials, those who try to keep up to date through continuing medical education or by being involved in professional college activities are more likely to be using better evidence than those who do neither of these. Be cautious about practitioners who rely only on their early university medical education or information from the pharmaceutical industry.

Does your practitioner share information with you?

Another important issue is whether your practitioner's decision-making process is based on sharing information with you – whether it be about the diagnosis, prognosis or intervention options.

A few years ago, one of us (Judy) developed a very severe pain and restricted movement in one shoulder, and was diagnosed with a tear in one of the ligaments in the rotator cuff and some tendon impingement. (This means the tendon had been 'pinched' or compressed slightly by the swelling.) When the pain persisted after some analgesic treatment and a steroid injection, she saw a surgeon who had an exemplary decision-making process. He explained the possible causes and implications of Judy's condition, and then told her the options and their risks and benefits. He also gave her some written information to take home to read.

Her options, as he explained them, were:

- Watchful waiting: he said that, according to published studies, the pain was likely to ease within a year or so, if nothing was done.
- Arthroscopic repair: he said that studies show most people report considerable relief after surgical repair by arthroscopy, a relatively simple procedure to remove the impingement. But Judy remained cautious because these were case studies based on personal testimony and therefore it was not clear whether the

improvement was a result of the intervention or would have occurred anyway. It is also possible that those in whom the operation was unsuccessful were not included in these reports.

• A more complicated surgical procedure: this option, he explained, would repair the ligament and increase the rotator cuff mobility. It would require a few days in hospital and intensive, prolonged physiotherapy.

Does your practitioner take account of your preferences?

On the basis of Judy's discussion with the surgeon and the written information that he provided, she decided that the potential harms of surgery, although small in her case, were sufficient to outweigh the potential benefits – which seemed unclear anyway. In addition, as she is not an athlete and not heavily reliant on the use of her shoulder, Judy could afford the time to wait and watch.

For some time afterwards, the pain woke Judy at night, making her question the wisdom of her choice. But within several months, she was almost completely pain free and after a few more months, she regained the mobility in her shoulder. If the problem had continued, she might have reconsidered other options.

In fact the problem did recur several years later. For some months Judy tried to ignore the pain, hoping that it might resolve, but when it continued to get worse she went to see her practitioner. As she is averse to surgery, she asked about other options and he suggested physiotherapy with someone who has special expertise in shoulder problems. Judy decided to try that option on the grounds that it might help and was unlikely to do any harm – aside from the time and financial cost that she felt were reasonable 'harms'. The physiotherapist gave her a regimen of stretching and strengthening exercises that he monitored regularly and adapted as Judy's mobility increased. Within a week or two she noticed a dramatic improvement, suggesting that the physiotherapy was working. Judy continues with a maintenance programme of exercise every other day, which she tries to adhere to, but, when she lapses for a week or two, some stiffness and discomfort return. It seems to her that the physiotherapy is doing the trick, as judged by criteria outlined in Chapter 8.

In contrast to Judy's experience, a friend, Sarah, who had a similar problem with her shoulder, had an unpleasant experience with her practitioner. He had diagnosed inflammation in the rotator cuff, but had not dealt with her concerns in the same caring way that Judy's had done. He had dismissed her questions saying 'Anything I haven't already told you is not important.'

After speaking with Judy, she decided to go back to her practitioner and ask for more information. She was nervous about doing this, and was worried that he might be upset or resentful at her questioning – after all, it is not always easy for a patient to question their doctor, and doctors are not always used to being closely questioned.

But it was much easier than Sarah expected. Once she'd clearly and calmly explained her concerns and her wish for more information, her doctor provided the information and she decided that the potential benefits of surgery outweighed the small risks. Her lifestyle – having a small child and a job that involved using her arms a great deal – was not conducive to waiting it out as Judy had done. Her choice to undergo surgery was driven by personal preferences relating to her lifestyle.

Judging a practitioner's technical expertise

After you and your practitioner have decided either to treat or to investigate your illness further, the procedure should be done by someone with the appropriate technical ability.

> The degree of expertise of any surgeon is extremely difficult for either a GP or a patient to assess. Surgeons who enjoy a high media profile may, in fact, be more competent at issuing press releases than at performing surgery.
>
> *Guy Maddern*[4]

To assist you in judging whether your practitioner has the necessary technical expertise, you might want to know whether he or she:
* is qualified to perform the procedure
* performs the procedure often enough
* is part of a quality assurance scheme or some similar programme.

If you are seeing a practitioner in a large outpatient's department or clinic, ask who will be performing the procedure. If it is not the practitioner whom you are consulting, ask the same questions about the person who will be doing the procedure. In some settings it may be a trainee, in which case you also need to know who will be supervising the trainee and something about the supervisor's experience.

Is your practitioner qualified to perform the procedure?

Among the issues that you should consider are the practitioner's special qualifications or certification to undertake this particular procedure. Even for a relatively minor operation such as an arthroscopic repair for a shoulder injury, you are likely to be better off choosing a surgeon specialising in shoulders. An unsupervised surgeon who is inexperienced in the procedure will not be a wise choice.

Report cards on doctors or health services have been discussed as an option but there is debate about how reliable they are. Some professional colleges have membership databases that will help you find a surgeon in a particular location who operates within a particular specialty area such as breast surgery (www.surgeons.org). Other directories are available, such as mydr.com.au, but none of these provides sufficient detail about the credentials of the doctor concerned. Websites based in the USA will provide you with a report card on a particular doctor for a fee. In the USA, patients tend not to use the report cards but rather follow the advice of their referring doctor. Even the former US President, Bill Clinton, went to one of the lowest-rated hospitals for heart surgery despite the publicly available rating. In addition to this, it has been shown that some hospitals tend to 'fudge' the reports by selecting 'safe' patients for their reporting framework. Doctor and hospital report cards appear to need more work if they are to become useful tools for patients and other interested parties.

How often does your practitioner perform the procedure?

It is useful to know how many of the particular procedures your practitioner does in a week, month or year – depending on how common the procedure is. There is evidence that patients are more likely to have better outcomes after a procedure if their doctors perform many such procedures.[5,6] Centres that specialise in a particular condition are also more likely to offer comprehensive, multidisciplinary care. But there is a paradox: although experience may increase with age, physical and mental agility decline. Professor Guy Maddern,[4] an eminent Australian surgeon, notes that many hospitals now recommend that surgeons should not operate after the age of 70:

> While clearly some surgeons could go on longer than this and others should have stopped much earlier, choosing a surgeon over 70 to perform your operation is perhaps ill-advised.

Is your practitioner part of a quality assurance scheme?

The third important criterion for assessing technical competence is whether your practitioner belongs to a quality assurance or credentialing scheme to assess technical proficiency. This will be relevant only to major interventions, such as surgery. Quality assurance schemes monitor patient care by examining patient records at random to make sure that care adheres to established practice, by monitoring adverse outcomes and by evaluating satisfaction through patient surveys. Many hospitals also have a credentialing process, to ensure that practitioners are appropriately qualified and skilled to undertake certain procedures. To ensure that a practitioner is covered by such a programme, you could ask the practitioner directly, your referring practitioner or the hospital.

All doctors are required to participate in continuing education programmes with their respective professional college and this is now a mandatory condition of registration. For most other health professions this is optional.

Many people ask whether litigation is a measure of a practitioner's technical competence, assuming that those who have been sued are best avoided. However, we do not believe that this is a reliable indicator of technical competence because studies have shown that litigation often reflects poor communication between practitioner and patient rather than technical failings

Finding a practice or hospital that suits your needs

Apart from looking for an evidence-based practitioner with good clinical expertise, there may be practical issues that you want to consider. These might include the location of the practice or hospital near your home or work, the gender of the doctors at the practice, the hours of opening and after-hours arrangements, the fee structure and any special expertise among the practitioners such as an interest in skin cancers or young families or women's health.

Choosing not to choose

You might feel unable to participate actively in decision-making if you are overwhelmed by serious illness or have other problems. In this case, you also have the right to delegate decision-making.

But think hard about this. The more serious your health problem, the more valuable your participation is likely to be. So, if you do find yourself wanting to delegate decision-making to your practitioner, and if the problem does not require immediate attention, take some time out. Arrange to see your practitioner again after you have had a chance to reflect.

If you decide to delegate decision-making, your practitioner will be better able to make informed decisions if he or she knows something about your preferences, your general attitude and your lifestyle. It may also be a good idea to ensure that a friend or relative is aware of your health preferences in case the need arises.

Summary

Everyone who offers you health advice should not only respect your right to be involved, but also encourage your participation. If you feel it necessary, ask for written information to take home with you.

- In most situations, you should expect your practitioner to explain to you:
  - what your problem is thought to be
  - what you can reasonably expect if your illness or condition is not treated
  - the benefits and harms of the various treatment and diagnostic test options.

- When choosing a practitioner, you should consider whether they:
  - are abreast of the latest evidence from randomised controlled trials
  - share information with you
  - respect your involvement in decision-making.

- If you are considering having a procedure, you should also assess the practitioner's technical competence by asking about:
  - their qualifications
  - how often they do the procedure
  - whether they are part of a quality assurance programme.

References

1. Davey H, Barratt A, Davey E et al. Medical tests: women's reported and preferred decision-making roles and preferences for information on benefits, side-effects and false results. *Health Expect* 2002;**5**:330–40.
2. Coulter A, Jenkinson C. European patients' views of the responsiveness of health systems and healthcare providers. *Eur J Public Hlth* 2005;**15**:355–60.
3. UK Department of Health. *Better information, better choices, better health: putting information at the centre of health.* 2004. http://www.dh.gov.uk/en/Publicationsandstatistics/Publications/PublicationsPolicyAndGuidance/DH_4098576
4. Maddern G. *Questions You Should Ask Your Surgeon.* Sydney: Bay Books, 1994.
5. Begg C, Cramer L, Hoskins W, Brennan M. Impact of hospital volume on operative mortality for major cancer surgery. *JAMA* 1998;**280**:1747–51.
6. Hannan E, Racz M, Ryan T. Coronary angioplasty volume–outcome relationships for hospitals and cardiologists. *JAMA* 1995;**277**:892–8.

III

Stories and studies

7

An education in shopping

Earlier in this book, we discussed the smart health choice essentials, five questions for deciding how best to deal with a health problem. They are:

1. What will happen if I wait and watch?
2. What are my test or treatment options?
3. What are the benefits and harms of these options?
4. How do the benefits and harms weigh up for me?
5. Do I have enough information to make a choice?

This section deals with what to do if the answer to the last question is that you do not have enough information to make a choice. Sometimes this situation can arise if you have been given conflicting information, perhaps because different practitioners are citing different research results. A lot of poor quality research is used as a basis for what is sometimes euphemistically called evidence. Be warned that poor studies can provide evidence that is, at best, weak and, at worst, dangerously misleading.

In the shopping centre ...

As Jenny guided her trolley along the aisle, she heard a familiar voice coming from the other side of the cereals. It was her cousin, Elise, chatting to someone.

'... Celbequine, Jack. Wonderful for arthritis too. It's really worked for my tennis elbow.... And it's completely natural so it can't do any harm. Just herbs and vitamins. It's been scientifically proven to cure people.'

'Is that so eh? Maybe I should try it. My leg's really been playing up lately. So where do I get it? How much does it cost?'

'To be honest, Jack, it's not cheap. But I look at this way:

'Three months' supply costs the same as a visit to my physio. Look, I've got a brochure here, tells you exactly how it works. It says: "Stimulates the body's own immune system with a combination of herbs and vitamins and helps to relieve pain. Contains extracts of celery and barley, calcium, beta-carotene, vitamin A, vitamin D .... Research shows that this blend of powerful ingredients prevents cartilage loss and slows down the progression of arthritis." It also says: "May cause nausea, stomach pain or diarrhoea."

Anyway, it works for me.'

Jack thanked Elise and promised to think about the tablets.

Jenny continued her shopping, thinking about what she had just overheard. It was something she often thought about: how easy it is to convince people that something works by describing how it is supposed to work. In her 8 years as a practitioner she had come across this phenomenon all too often. And not just with her patients – she had seen many pharmaceutical company representatives use similar arguments when trying to convince her to prescribe their products.

Now Jenny happened to know Jack, and she was worried that he might buy the tablets, which she knew he could not afford, having recently been laid off work. It occurred to her that the pain in his leg might not even be caused by arthritis; it could be sciatic pain arising from an old back injury. In addition, he had previously undergone surgery for a stomach ulcer, which meant that he may be at high risk of suffering the tablets' side effect of stomach irritation. In short, Jenny knew that, even if these tablets did relieve Jack's leg pain, the harms might outweigh the benefit.

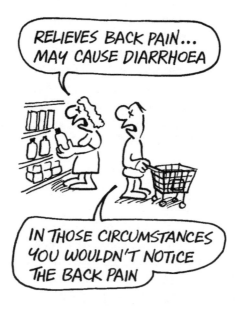

Jenny bumped into Elise in the next aisle, and invited her for a coffee after they'd finished shopping.

How believable are the claims? ...

Later, over coffee, Jenny admitted overhearing some of the conversation with Jack, and asked about the brochure's claim that a trial reported 130 people were helped by the tablets. 'But do they tell you how many people were treated altogether?'

'Not that I recall,' said Elise. 'But why do you ask?'

'Well, if 150 people were treated and 130 improved, that's pretty good. But if thousands were treated and only 130 improved, it's a different matter. That means a lot of people took tablets for no benefit, yet risking the known side effects, not to mention those that are not yet known. It's important to know, not just how many got better, but how many were treated.'

Elise was intrigued: 'I get what you're saying, Jen, but the fact of the matter is that I felt better on those tablets, so they obviously work.'

'There are many reasons why you could be feeling better. You might just have improved anyway, which happens more often with health problems than many people realise. And people tend to feel better when they have taken some positive action, even if the action itself has no effect. The point is, when health claims are made about any product, the research supporting these claims must be valid and the potential benefits and harms should be clearly described so consumers can make an informed choice.'

About the trial ...

After Jenny had seen her last patient later that day, she found Elise in her waiting room. Elise had rung the manufacturer to find out more about the trial, and was excited by the results. The 130 helped by the treatment were out of a group of 250, and the manufacturer said this meant about 50 per cent of people could expect to improve on the treatment. This is how the research was described to Elise:

> During the first week of the opening of a new mall, free samples of Celbequine were handed out to shoppers who said they had joint pain or arthritis. Each sample of 25 tablets was enough for one week's treatment, after which the shoppers were invited to re-order free supplies each month over a 6-month period. At the end of 5 months, there were still 525 people in the trial. They were asked to fill in a questionnaire to receive their final quota of free tablets. A competition offering a prize of gym membership was included with the questionnaire.

What transpired was that only 250 of the 525 questionnaires were completed and returned. Out of these, 130 indicated 'considerable improvement' within 6 months of starting the treatment. Elise calcu-lated that 130 out of 250 meant about a 50 per cent follow-up rate, as stated by the manufacturer.

But Jenny was not so sure. 'These figures could be important, but I'm still sceptical. First, you have to understand that pain from arthritis – or from many conditions for that matter – is not constant.

It often fluctuates. Many of my patients with arthritis have long periods relatively pain free. They just improve spontaneously without any treatment.'

Jenny scribbled some figures as she continued: 'They told you 130 people got better out of 250 who filled out the question-naires. What about the other 275 people? Maybe they couldn't be bothered to fill out the forms because they thought the treatment useless? You can see what will happen if we include them in the calculations.'

'Yes,' said Elise. 'It might mean that only 130 out of 525 got better. That's ... less than 25 per cent who felt any benefit. But, wait a minute, what if it worked the other way? What if the people who didn't respond did feel some improvement but were then less likely to fill in the forms because they weren't so conscious of their aches? That could mean that three-quarters of people felt some benefit. But how do we know which is correct?'

'That's the point exactly,' said Jenny. 'We don't know. It's very difficult to draw any firm conclusions from this sort of study. Suppose the prize of gym membership influenced who was likely to send in the form. What if it meant that people who were feeling fit and well were more likely to send it back? Or you could argue the other way: that the healthier, fitter people are less likely to be interested in such a prize because they already go to the gym. Either way, you could argue that the study was more likely to include certain types of people. This is what researchers call selection bias, and makes it difficult to know whether the treatment really works.'

Elise interrupted: 'So what you're really saying is that we don't know whether the tablets made 25 per cent of people feel better or 75 per cent of people feel better?'

'And we don't even know that,' continued Jenny. 'Remember that many hundreds more people, maybe even thousands, were given samples. Why did all those other people drop out of the survey? Maybe they suffered stomach pains or other side effects. Again, this is selection bias. As we don't know what happened to everyone in the trial, we have no way of knowing whether the tablets worked.'

Some things get better on their own ...

Jenny could see that much of this was new to Elise. She wanted to finish her train of thought, so she went on: 'There is a very important phenomenon that is often overlooked. Researchers call it spontaneous remission, but all it means is that, in many instances, time heals. Our bodies have a marvellous capacity for recovery. For a lot of conditions, people get better without any treatment.

'So getting back to the question of whether there is good evidence that Celbequine is effective: how do we know if the people who reported improvement were responding to these tablets or perhaps to something else that they were taking, or whether the pain just got better on its own, which might have happened even without Celbequine? Don't forget that these are people who were well enough to be walking around a shopping centre when the trial began, which means their symptoms may not have been too bad to start off with. If that was the case, there's a good chance they may have recovered on their own, with no treatment at all.'

The placebo effect ...

Reaching for a book from the shelf, Jenny continued: 'Now there's something else that often gets in the way when you're trying to judge the effects of a treatment. Let me read you something from this book by Norman Cousins called *Anatomy of an Illness as Perceived by the Patient*. It's a marvellous account of how he dealt with a very serious disease in a most unconventional way.

'This is the part where he's describing a placebo:

"A striking example of the doctor's role in making a placebo work can be seen in an experiment in which patients with bleeding ulcers were divided into two groups. Members of the first group were informed by the doctor that a new drug had just been developed that would undoubtedly produce relief. The second group was told by the nurses that a new experimental drug would be administered, but that very little was known about its effects. Seventy per cent of the people in the first group received sufficient relief from their ulcers. Only 25 per cent of the patients in the second group experienced similar benefit. Both groups had been given the identical 'drug' – a placebo." [1]

Elise thought for a moment. 'So the implication is that the people in the trial could have been improving just because they were told they would – because they believed the tablets worked.'

'Yes, there's certainly the strong possibility that some were responding to the placebo effect,' said Jenny. 'The mind has mysterious powers. Sometimes believing is seeing! The placebo effect is very helpful but we want to know whether an intervention that has some risks and costs has an effect over and above its placebo effect.'

And other study flaws ...

'And there's another problem with the way that this study was done. Having accepted free samples of the product, I bet not many people could have said it did absolutely nothing to make them feel better, let alone that it made them feel sick. I'm not saying people deliberately lie, but there's often a temptation to be more positive than one might genuinely be feeling. This is sometimes called "acquiescence bias" and is an example of measurement bias. Imagine you're in the supermarket and you're offered a sample slice of a lemon meringue pie that you accept. The salesperson asks how you like it, with one of those smiles that says "isn't it just too delicious for words". Many people would find it difficult to say otherwise.

'So getting back to the questionnaires, we've seen there could be several biases: one in the way people interpret and report their health outcomes, called measurement bias, and another in the exclusion of who knows how many hundreds of people who originally entered the trial – selection bias. The bottom line is that there is still no sound evidence that Celbequine does more good than harm.'

Elise was a little hesitant: 'I follow what you've said, Jen, but are you telling me there is absolutely no value in the testimonies of those 130 people who thought the treatment helped them?'

'What I'm saying is that when you're making an important decision about whether some treatment is effective or not, your judgement should be based on stronger evidence than the personal testimonies of just a few people who took the intervention. This is true whether you're a researcher doing a study on the effect of an intervention, or a consumer, or a practitioner advising a patient.'

Personal experiences can be important . . .

'But your question is valid. Are anecdotes based on personal experience ever valuable? The answer is most certainly yes. If you experience a dramatic, immediate change in your symptoms after some treatment for a condition that usually lasts a long time without any treatment, and you experience the same, strong, rapid effect on several subsequent occasions, then your experience provides evidence of the treatment working for you. Let's say, for example, you have regular migraine attacks that usually last several hours and a new tablet stops the pain within half an hour every time you take it. There's little doubt the tablet is working, for you anyway. But for most medications, the effects are not that dramatic. For most medications, the improvements we are looking for are more subtle and occur over a longer period. This is where individuals' reports are of little value.

'Getting back to Celbequine; the information said it would take up to 6 months to work and also said something about retarding the development of arthritis long term. So in this case, individual reports are not a reliable guide to its efficacy. Remember that individual reports of improvement are no more than that – reports of how people feel after treatment. They do not tell us anything about what may have caused the improvement – whether it was the treatment, something else happening in the person's life or just the passage of time.

'Individual reports are of little use when we want to know what some medium-term or long-term change is caused by. That's another story entirely. To make this kind of deduction, we need probabilistic data, that is, information about the percentage of people who improved. Moreover, we need to compare this percentage with the percentage who would have improved without the treatment.'

Let's get sceptical ...

Jenny continued slowly and deliberately: 'So the marketers of Celbequine might have done themselves a favour – if their product truly is as good as they claim – by doing their homework before embarking on a costly bit of research that was clearly full of weaknesses. On the other hand, if their claims are unwarranted, they might not want people to know. At the end of the day, if a product's claims are genuine, well-designed research can only strengthen the claims, whereas, if there is no valid evidence to back their claims, we should remain sceptical.

'To make well-informed choices about important decisions that may affect our health – our bodies and our minds – we need much more than opinions. We need evidence.'

They were both silent for a moment, then Jenny said: 'But if you want my opinion, I think it's time to call it a day!'

From detergents to treatment for acne ...

When they met again a few days later, Elise was excited as she described her investigations of a new detergent that had been advertised as a breakthrough in 'enzymatic power' that 'gets whites whiter than white'.

As it was more expensive than her regular powder, Elise wanted to test the claim. She divided her whites into two, and used her regular detergent for one load and the new product on the other.

'And then I thought that this is the way that Celbequine should have been tested,' she said. 'Get two groups of people with the same health problem; give one group the treatment and give the others nothing or the old treatment.'

'Bravo,' said Jenny. 'You've hit the nail on the head. But to take it a step further, imagine that you were setting up a study for a new acne treatment. What would you do?'

'You need a bunch of people with acne,' replied Elise. 'Teenagers. You could approach high schools or advertise in teenage magazines asking for volunteers. And then divide them into two groups. One group is given the treatment and the other ... what do they get? I mean what's in it for the volunteers if they're not getting the new treatment?'

'Good point,' said Jenny. 'What say we tell the teenagers that we're testing a new acne lotion. We don't know whether it works or not but you could help us find out by taking part in a trial. The trial will work like this: we spin a coin – heads, you get the treatment, tails you get some other lotion that looks, feels, smells like the treatment but is inert, a placebo. If the new treatment is shown to work, we will offer a free course of treatment at the end of the trial to everyone who was given the placebo.

'Doing it this way, you see, excludes other variables that might affect the outcome. For instance, the massaging action of applying the cream might do some good – or some bad for that matter.'

Elise was hooked. 'And remember what you read me about the placebo effect? If the volunteers aren't told whether they're getting the treatment or placebo, this will stop their expectations influencing the results. No measurement bias, right?'

Randomised and blinded . . .

'Right! And there's another thing. In a comparative study, it's essential that the groups are similar if you want the results to be valid. A good way to ensure this is to allocate the treatment randomly. You've heard of randomised controlled trials, haven't you? Well, randomisation addresses the possibility that those who did not get the treatment were sicker than those who did – or vice versa. Randomisation, or random allocation as it is sometimes called, can be done by the toss of a coin, or by other techniques – computers can be used to allocate patients randomly to a treatment or placebo.

'Each volunteer is randomly allocated to the new treatment or to the placebo; in addition, as you've already said, people shouldn't know what group they're in. In other words, they should be masked or "blinded" to whether they are getting the treatment or placebo. This is the way drug licensing authorities assess new claims about the effects of drugs.'

The two women sat in thought for a while. Then Jenny went on:

'Listen Elise, obviously you and I can't rush off and do a randomised controlled trial on every new pill or powder on the market, but the healthcare system is continuously involved in studies of all types. There are researchers out there doing randomised controlled trials all the time ... or RCTs as they are sometimes called. What consumers should be doing, however, is asking their practitioners for evidence supporting their recommendations about treatments or any tests – especially for important decisions. The onus is on the person or organisation that recommends the product or the treatment or the service to supply sound evidence that it improves or prolongs life. This includes practitioners from all areas and doctrines of healthcare, and the pharmaceutical companies who recommend their products.

'Thousands of studies are published every year – though not all of them are randomised controlled trials – and are accessible to practitioners either in journals or in summarised form on electronic databases. So when evidence is available, it should be used.'

Do the benefits outweigh the harms? ...

'If I were approached by representatives of this company to recommend Celbequine to my patients, I would expect them to provide me with sound evidence that my patients are going to be better off. Failing that, I could do a computerised search to see whether there is any evidence in the medical literature. I could find Medline on the internet, for example, and look at the abstracts of studies published in the most important journals in recent years. Or I could look up the Cochrane Library, which is a regularly updated electronic library of summaries of all the randomised controlled trials (see page 138). The point is that, if I have no valid evidence that the benefits of a treatment outweigh its harms, I should be careful about recommending it. Most practitioners now have access to online computer systems in their offices to search for valid evidence. Mind you, being available on the internet means it can be accessed by anyone.'

Elise thought for a bit. 'Why didn't the manufacturer do the study right in the first place?'

'Now that,' said Jenny, 'is a very interesting question. Maybe they don't know about randomised controlled trials or maybe they think consumers won't know the difference. It's just possible, of course, that the stuff doesn't work and they prefer not to make that knowledge public. Or maybe, good evidence is simply not available. After all, randomised trials can be complex and expensive to conduct.

So does it really work? . . .

'But let's get back to the question at hand: does Celbequine really work? The only information that we have is not very convincing because it is based on individual reports. This can be misleading for many reasons: first, people often improve spontaneously with time; second, they might be responding to the placebo effect. Of course, it could be that the treatment really does work. But we can't judge this from the information available. And yet we have this situation where expensive, potentially dangerous interventions are recommended without valid evidence that they work. What we need is good research to supply valid evidence so that all of us can make informed judgements about our health.'

Elise thanked her cousin and left with a mixture of new-found confidence as well as surprise that she had been so poorly informed before. Why, only a few days ago she would have thought herself as well informed as the next person. Then she realised, with some surprise, that she probably had been.

Note: the name 'Celbequine' is purely fictitious.

Reference

1. Cousins N. Anatomy of an Illness as Perceived by a Patient. UK: WW Norton & Co Ltd. 2005.

8

The weakness of one

Theists, for example, note the number of times their prayers have been answered and conclude that there is a benevolent god; atheists cite the occasions that their prayers have gone unanswered and conclude that we are on our own. Both need to develop the habit of thinking more broadly. Both must consider the number of times their hopes have been answered when they have prayed and when they have not, as well as the number of times their hopes have been dashed when they have prayed and when they have not

Thomas Gilovich[1]

One of the points raised in Chapter 7 is the compelling allure of personal testimony. For many of us, this is one of the most seductive sources of health information. A neighbour says her cancer disappeared after she took shark cartilage. Your mother swears that taking a vitamin C tablet every morning keeps her free of colds. A colleague claims his bad back recovered after doing a certain exercise for 6 weeks.

It can be tempting to draw conclusions from such anecdotes; somehow a story involving a real person whom you know can seem more convincing than the results of studies based on thousands of anonymous participants. Anecdotal evidence is usually based on individual experiences or observations, as distinct from probabilistic evidence that gives estimates of how likely something is to occur based on experience with large numbers of people. In this chapter we discuss some of the ways in which stories can be helpful in making health decisions, but also warn of their limitations.

The danger of the anecdote

There are inherent dangers in relying totally on anecdotes. Consider the case of Mr Dickens, 70, who recently consulted Dr Carter about an irregular pulse. Mr Dickens, who has previously had high blood pressure and a stroke, is found to have a disturbance of his heart rhythm, called atrial fibrillation. This condition may cause a blood clot to develop in the heart and send off fragments that can cause a stroke by blocking arteries in the brain. One treatment used in people with atrial fibrillation is an anticoagulant, which prevents a blood clot. But Dr Carter knows that this drug can also cause internal bleeding, with potentially serious consequences, although she has never had a patient suffer this particular side effect. After she prescribes the treatment, Mr Dickens has a bleed into the brain.

Soon after, Dr Carter sees Mr Jones, another elderly man with similar problems to Mr Dickens. But Dr Carter does not prescribe an anticoagulant this time, discouraged by her recent experience with Mr Dickens. Mr Jones later suffers a stroke. Dr Carter will never know if this might have been prevented if she had prescribed an anticoagulant. But an examination of the probabilistic evidence – as distinct from the anecdotal evidence provided by case reports – gives us some idea.

If Dr Carter had done a literature search, she would have found several good randomised controlled trials showing a two-thirds reduction in stroke for patients treated with anticoagulants. On the other hand, serious bleeds from anticoagulation are rare, so overall her patients with atrial fibrillation would be served best by taking anticoagulants unless they are at low risk of stroke or at high risk of bleeding. Mr Dickens is at high risk of stroke because he has high blood pressure and has had a previous stroke. Out of 1000 people like Mr Dickens who are treated, about 120 strokes would be prevented in the next year, whereas a bleed into the brain as a result of anticoagulants would occur in about 5 people. In addition, there may be other bleeding, some of which would be mainly a nuisance such as bruises, and some of which could be more serious, such as bleeds into the stomach or bowel.

> It [an anecdote] is useful for documenting that the outcome can occur, but provides no information about the frequency with which it occurs or the effect of an intervention on the frequency of occurrence.
>
> *David Eddy*[2]

Only survivors speak!

Anecdotes have limited use in judging the effectiveness of health interventions. If you wanted to know, for example, whether a certain cancer treatment saves lives, the opinion of someone who had the

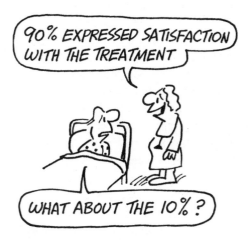

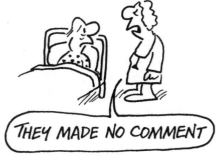

treatment would not be a reliable guide. Remember that those patients in whom the treatment did not work are no longer around to give their views. Only survivors speak – which can result in a very biased picture of an intervention.

More problems with anecdotes

Another problem with anecdotal experience is that we tend to give the most recent and negative experience undue bias. As a result of this phenomenon, most of us are inclined to be over-confident when making predictions based on a recent experience, even when we have more reliable probabilistic information on hand. It is therefore especially inadvisable to use anecdotal evidence to assess a treatment with long-term effects.

Here are the reasons why anecdotal evidence is weak when judging most interventions:

- The outcomes of most health problems are not predictable for any individual. How a health problem will affect an individual is difficult to predict and can be expressed only as a probability. For example, you may have a 40 per cent chance of surviving for another 10 years. An intervention can be judged only by the extent to which it changes this probability of survival. Just because you are alive at the end of 10 years does not mean that the intervention is responsible.
- The effects of most interventions are small and subtle. An intervention may increase the chance of living for 10 years from 40 per cent to 50 per cent. It would be impossible to detect such an improvement based on anecdotal reports.
- The effects of many interventions are long term. It is difficult to link an outcome – whether that happens to be a recurrence of disease, good health or death – to an intervention used years before. There may be a host of other factors involved.
- The effects of some interventions cannot be confirmed by testing the intervention on yourself again. If you suffer from migraine, which usually causes a persistent headache, and this symptom disappears as soon as you take a certain tablet, you

can test this hypothesis next time that you get a migraine. But most conditions do not recur repeatedly, so you have no opportunity for confirming the effect of an intervention.

But anecdotes can be useful in some situations

It is generally unwise to rely on other people's stories as a guide to how likely you are to experience similar benefits or harms from an intervention. However, anecdotes are useful in some situations.

When confronted by illness or other health problems, many people find it helpful to talk to others who have been through similar situations. Their stories can provide useful insights into how your life might be affected by a similar illness, or side effects from a treatment, and what strategies might be useful in helping you deal with them. Indeed, some universities now invite patients to talk to medical students about their own experiences with illness, in an attempt to ensure that doctors become more understanding of and sympathetic to what it is like to be a patient. Other people's stories can also provide useful information on how to find your way around the health system, which can seem like a confusing maze to a newcomer. Patient support groups can be particularly useful in these situations.

Most scientific and medical discoveries have their roots in anecdotes, which have led to hypotheses that are then proved by rigorous testing. In some circumstances, the anecdotal evidence can be so spectacularly convincing that the need for further confirmation diminishes. For example, when Howard Florey and Ernst Chain developed the drug penicillin based on Alexander Fleming's earlier work, the antibiotic properties were so striking that it was introduced for use without long-term trials. When people are treated for an illness and survive in the face of evidence that most people die without treatment, there is usually little doubt about the treatment's efficacy.

Let's explore a situation where personal experience may help to decide whether a treatment works. Consider the case of Ed Smith, who suffers from severe migraines. When a migraine strikes, Ed is incapacitated and has to lie down for several hours. He has tried many supposed remedies over the years, but none has worked. He hears from a friend about a new therapy that has helped her. He tries it the next time he feels a migraine starting, and his pain disappears quickly.

Is Ed's excitement about the treatment well founded? He knows that the pain disappeared quickly when he took the tablets, and that they helped his friend. He now also needs to know whether he will experience the same immediate benefit when he takes the tablets again. If indeed he tries it again and he experiences the same pain relief, he probably has good reason to feel excited.

As with the introduction of penicillin, anecdotal evidence can be used to assess the affect of a treatment if at least some of several principles are fulfilled:

- The outcome of the disease or condition is predictable in the absence of the treatment. The condition in question does not usually get better on its own, at least not immediately.
- The effect of the treatment is immediate. The outcome is evident soon after the treatment.
- The effect of the treatment is large. There is a dramatic, large and obvious effect that would be difficult to attribute to spontaneous improvement.
- The effect of the treatment can be confirmed by repetition. If the nature of the condition is such that it recurs, it is possible to confirm the treatment's effects by repeated testing.

Acting on someone else's anecdotal experience is appropriate only if the harm seems small and the benefit worthwhile. Suppose that you suffer from chapped, itchy skin in winter, and a friend tells you about a new cream that helped him. Should you try it? It sounds like you should. First, if it relieves the dryness and itch, you can be fairly sure the cream is responsible if previous treatments have failed to make any difference. Second, because treatment is likely to be short term, the risks of serious adverse effects are low. Third, judging whether the cream is effective is straightforward. So, if the cream works, you will benefit and, if it doesn't, you stand to lose very little.

N of 1 trials

We could be more scientific about assessing the effect of the anti-itch cream, even with just one person, by using what we call an 'N of 1' trial. These trials have been defined as:

> ... [a trial where] the patient undergoes pairs of treatment periods organised so that one period involves the use of experimental treatment and the other involves the use of an alternate or placebo therapy. The patient and physician are blinded, if possible, and outcomes are monitored. Treatment periods are replicated until the clinician and patient are convinced that the treatments are definitely different or definitely not different.

If we had a 'fake' or placebo cream as well as the active one and tried each, one at a time, without realising which one we had tried, this would be an 'N of 1' trial. Ed Smith could have done one of these for his migraine treatment if he did not have labels on the pills and tried the new one against a fake one without knowing which was which.

In short, anecdotal information is useful when you are looking for immediate symptomatic relief for a relatively minor condition, and there is little potential for the treatment to do harm. It is also useful if you want to know how other people coped with a specific problem, or gain some insight into their experiences of diseases or interventions. It might be helpful for generating hypotheses that can be more rigorously tested.

A broad range of stories

But what if we have a collection of stories on the same topic? This may help us to learn about the context of what can happen in an illness or the likely sequence of events.[3] For example, the same strain of flu can render one person sick in bed for a fortnight whereas another manages to keep functioning and is better within 4 or 5 days. People's stories can be used to develop concepts and hypotheses, which can then be more rigorously tested and evaluated with a large group of people and in different settings.

The usefulness of a broad range of stories depends on how they have been collected and analysed. On most topics, if you listen to enough people's stories, eventually you will start to hear similar accounts of the illness or treatment in question. As a very rough guide, this usually happens when you start to collect more than about 30 stories and you can be reasonably confident that you've captured the most common and likely experience of an illness or its treatment. Ideally two different researchers should look at recordings of the stories and identify the common themes within them.

A good example of this is a website called DiPEx (Database of Individual Patients' Experience) at www.dipex.org. This website has over 100 modules on different illnesses and patient experiences. Each module consists of a number of patients' stories that typify over 40 or 50 stories that were recorded on each topic. This means that the main patient experiences are more likely to be covered.

A resource like this is more powerful and useful than just one anecdote when you are trying to make a decision, because it is a bit more balanced and provides a range of experiences from a number of people, not just one perspective or opinion. However, although it gives a range of experiences, it does not provide information on how commonly they occur.

Summary

As seductive as anecdotal reports can be, it is usually unwise to rely on generalisations based on one or two experiences. They do not tell us the most probable outcome, which is most useful for guiding decisions. Anecdotal evidence is useful to help you understand the nature of the symptoms of a disease and of the side effects of treatment. However, anecdotes are poor evidence of how likely that outcome is to occur, except in a few circumstances as shown below:

continued

Table 8.1 Comparison between reliable and unreliable use of anecdotal evidence

Anecdotal evidence is reliable	Anecdotal evidence is unreliable
When the outcomes of the disease or condition are predictable in the absence of treatment (e.g. migraines, chronic arthritic pain, premenstrual tension)	When the outcomes of the treatment are uncertain for the individual (e.g. breast cancer, diabetes)
When the effects of the treatment are large	When the effects of the treatment are small and subtle
When the effects of the treatment are immediate	When the effects of the treatment are delayed
When the effects of treatment can be confirmed by repetition	When the effects of the treatment cannot be confirmed by repetition
When the effects of treatment can be confirmed by an 'N of 1' trial	When the effects of treatment are disproved by an 'N of 1' trial

References

1. Gilovich T. *How We Know What Isn't So: the fallibility of human reason in everyday life.* New York: Free Press, 1991: 187.
2. Eddy D. A*ssessing Health Practices and Designing Practice Policies.* USA: American College of Physicians, 1992.
3. Greenhalgh T. *What Seems to be the Trouble? Stories in illness and healthcare.* Oxford: Radcliffe, 2006.

9

The power of many

... while the individual man is an insoluble puzzle, in the aggregate he becomes a mathematical certainty. You can, for example, never foretell what any man will do, but you can say with precision what an average number will be up to. Individuals vary, but percentages remain constant. So says the statistician.

Sir Arthur Conan Doyle[1]

The power of probabilities

We live in an uncertain world where, as is so often said, the only certainties are death and taxes. Even so, learning to ask the right questions can help reduce the uncertainties that surround health outcomes.

One of the important questions relates to the probability of events, such as the chances that an intervention will cause a particular benefit or harm. Although anecdotal evidence is generally unreliable because it is based on an individual's experience, probabilistic evidence is more reliable because it is based on the experiences of many and therefore tells you what is likely to happen. Probabilistic information is derived from studies involving many people. When assessing the probable outcome of a test or treatment, the most reliable probabilistic information comes from *randomised controlled trials* (RCTs) or *systematic reviews* of RCTs.

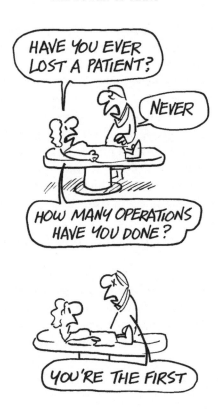

Probabilities – what do they tell us?

When making a decision about how to manage any health problem, probabilistic evidence answers the following questions:

1. How likely is a particular outcome?
2. What factors affect the chance of this happening?
3. How will a particular test or treatment change the chance of this happening?

How likely is a particular outcome?

To estimate how probable an event is, numbers are far better than verbal assurances or clichés. Suppose you are trying to assess the chances that a healthy 5 year old will suffer complications after a tonsillectomy. If your practitioner's response is 'I've never lost a patient from tonsillectomy' or 'the risks are small', you need to ask for probabilistic information. After all, what your practitioner considers a 'small risk' may be an unacceptable risk to you.

Far better to avoid misunderstandings through the use of data such as: 'one in 100 people has severe pain after this procedure' or 'one in 1000 people will need further surgery' or 'one in 100,000 people dies from this procedure'. If you are not given probabilistic data, ask for it. And if you do not understand what the figures mean, ask for them to be explained in terms that you do understand.

What factors affect the chance of this happening?

Many women are worried about their risk of developing breast cancer. Suppose that you hear on the news that the latest figures show that 91 in every 1000 women are at risk of breast cancer (that is, 1 in 11).[2] This sounds alarming. However, remember that a woman's age has a powerful effect on her risk of developing breast cancer at a particular time.

It has been estimated, for example, that 13 in every 1000 Australian women will develop breast cancer between the ages of 40 and 50, compared with 24 in every 1000 women between the ages of 60 and 70.[3] For breast cancer, another important risk factor – so named because it increases a woman's chance of developing the disease – is having a strong family history of the disease. Although women without such factors are at lesser risk of developing the disease, this does not mean that they are risk free. And, conversely, women with many risk factors for the disease will not necessarily develop it.

Being older affects people's risk in many situations. For example, elderly people are more likely to suffer serious complications from influenza than younger people. This is one of the reasons why annual flu immunisation is recommended for elderly people.

When making health decisions, you need to know what factors affect the probability of you having a particular outcome – whether it changes your chance of suffering nasty effects from a disease, test or treatment. Such factors could include your age, and your medical and family history.

Will a particular test or treatment change the chance of this happening to me?

The only way to find out whether a test or treatment will change the likelihood of an outcome is to turn to the results of studies that have compared the outcomes of people who received the test or treatment with the outcomes of those who did not.

It is this sort of study that tells us that children who have a persistent green runny nose will be more likely to recover if they have 10 days of antibiotics than those who do not. A Cochrane systematic review of six randomised controlled trials involving a total of 401 children recorded the number of children who were cured after randomly allocating some to receive antibiotics and the others to receive placebo pills.[4] No-one knew whether they were in the intervention or placebo group.

After finishing their course of tablets, 56 in 100 of the placebo group still had runny noses, compared with 40 in 100 of the antibiotic group. However, 2 in 100 children who were taking the placebo tablets reported side effects compared with a slightly higher 5 in 100 on the antibiotics.

Clearly, this study does not show that giving children antibiotics for persistently runny noses guarantees that they will be cured, but it increases the probability that they will. As we learnt earlier in this book, you might also have noticed that a fair number of children will get better without antibiotics too.

To find out more about how the effects of treatment are represented numerically, see Chapter 18 describing relative risk and risk difference.

Putting probabilities to work

Example 1: Anticoagulants for atrial fibrillation

Let's return to the example of Dr Carter from Chapter 8. Dr Carter's patient was an elderly man with atrial fibrillation (a disturbance of heart rhythm), and she was considering treating him with anticoagulants, which prevent blood clots forming. But Dr Carter also knew that anticoagulants can cause internal bleeding, so she had a dilemma. What a practitioner in her situation should do is to find out the probability of preventing a stroke by treating with anticoagulants, as well as the probability of serious side effects from anticoagulants.

If she had searched the medical literature, she would have found the following probabilistic information produced by the American College of Chest Physicians.

What is the probability that an elderly person with atrial fibrillation will have a stroke?

One option is not to take any medication for atrial fibrillation. Without medication, an average patient with atrial fibrillation (not caused by rheumatic fever) has about a 5 per cent chance of suffering a stroke in the following year (10 per cent over 2 years).[5]

What factors affect the probability of an elderly person with atrial fibrillation having a stroke?

As for most diseases, there are certain characteristics or risk factors that help to determine who is more likely and who is less likely to have a stroke in this situation. In this case, the risk of stroke increases with age, high blood pressure, some heart failure and any previous history of 'funny turns' or strokes. For example, if you are aged under 65 years and have none of the above risk factors, the chance of you having a stroke over the next 2 years is 2 in 100. This can be shown diagrammatically by the 100 faces in Figure 9.1: 98 of them do not have a stroke, one has a mild stroke (light shaded) and one has a severe stroke (darker shaded).

On the other hand, someone who is over the age of 75 years and has atrial fibrillation, and who also has high blood pressure, has a much higher risk of stroke over the next 2 years – 20 out of 100. Figure 9.2 shows this graphically.

Will anticoagulants change the probability of a stroke?

The answer is yes. Randomised controlled trials have shown that thinning the blood with either aspirin or the stronger drug

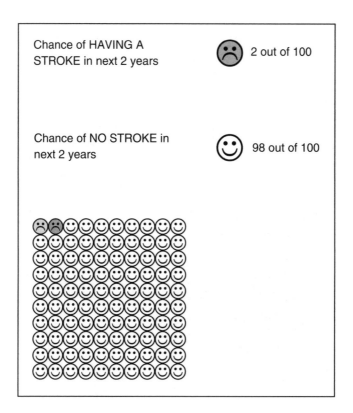

Figure 9.1 From *Making choices: treatments to prevent strokes in patients with atrial fibrillation.*[6] *(Light grey = minor stroke, dark grey = major stroke)*

warfarin can reduce the chance of stroke in people with atrial fibrillation. The risk of stroke is reduced by about 65 per cent with warfarin and by about 22 per cent with aspirin. This is because blood clots can form in the fibrillating heart chamber, break off and go up to the brain, causing a stroke. The higher your risk from the outset, the greater your benefit from treatment. A 65 per cent reduction if your risk starts out at 20 in 100 is going to mean it comes down to about 7 in 100, whereas if your risk of stroke starts out at 2 in 100 then warfarin will reduce it by 65 per cent to around 1 in 100.

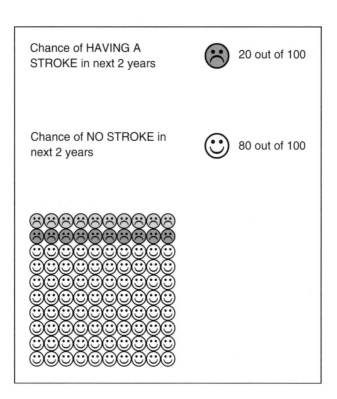

Figure 9.2 From *Making choices: treatments to prevent strokes in patients with atrial fibrillation.*[6] *(Light grey = minor stroke, dark grey = major stroke)*

However, it's not all good news because thinning the blood in this way also increases your chance of bleeding, which can be serious if it comes from a stomach ulcer or your brain, for instance. The chance of serious bleeding when taking warfarin is about 4 in 100 people. So, it's a trade-off between lowering your risk of stroke (bearing in mind how great your risk is from the outset if you do nothing) and your risk of stroke. Warfarin lowers your stroke risk by a greater amount but is more likely to cause serious bleeding. It seems that, in this case, as in most of life, you don't get something for nothing!

Any benefit of anticoagulants is 'bought' at a cost of an increased chance of a life-threatening bleed such as a stomach bleed (shown as black shading in Figure 9.3), in addition to minor bleeding such as

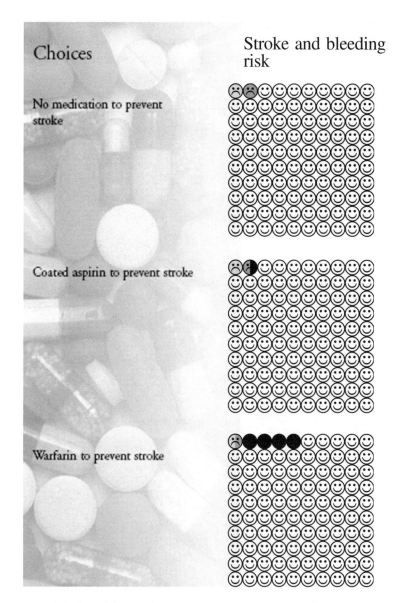

Figure 9.3 From *Making choices: treatments to prevent strokes in patients with atrial fibrillation.*[6] Version for people with low stroke risk. (Light grey = minor stroke, dark grey = major stroke, black = serious bleeding)

bruises, as well as the inconvenience and concern associated with the regular blood monitoring that is part of anticoagulant treatment. This price may be too high for some people, for example, someone who has

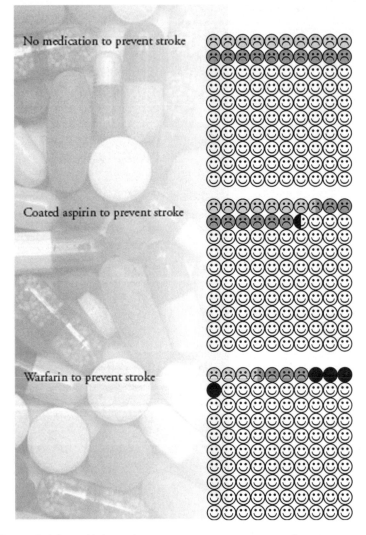

Figure 9.4 From *Making choices: treatments to prevent strokes in patients with atrial fibrillation.*[6] Version for people with high stroke risk. (Light grey = minor stroke, dark grey = major stroke, black = serious bleeding)

no risk factors for stroke, in whom taking anticoagulants will reduce his or her chance of stroke from 2 per cent to 1 per cent.

But for someone with all three risk factors for stroke, the price is likely to be outweighed by the benefit of reducing the chance of a stroke from 20 per cent to 7 per cent (Figure 9.4).

Aided by our practitioners, we need to exercise judgement in deciding how to apply probabilistic evidence to our own decision-making. For example, if you have atrial fibrillation and are at high risk of a stroke, anticoagulants are probably a good idea because the benefits outweigh the potential harms. But if you are at low risk of stroke, and especially if you have a high risk of bleeding, antico-agulants may be best avoided because the harms outweigh the benefits. If your risk is moderate, and the risks and benefits are less clear-cut, individual preferences become particularly important. The critical factor to consider here is how the individual weighs the 'value' of preventing a stroke against risking a bleed and other disad-vantages of taking anticoagulants, including the tendency to bleed and the need for regular monitoring.

The figures used to illustrate these probabilities come from a Canadian decision aid that is based on high-quality randomised controlled trials. It has four different versions, depending on your risk and can be found at www.canadianstrokenetwork/research/clinicians.php

Example 2: Hormone therapy after the menopause

Another common example where the probabilistic evidence needs to be carefully weighed is the use of hormone replacement therapy (HRT) after the menopause. In this case, women need to weigh up the short-term benefit of symptom relief from hot flushes and night sweats, against the longer-term risks of breast cancer, abnormal mammograms, blood clots and strokes. There also appears to be an increase in risk of heart attack during the first year of taking HRT.

As we mentioned earlier in this book, the results of a large well-conducted randomised controlled trial, the Women's Health Initiative (WHI), were published in 2003 and overturned some of our previous beliefs about HRT.[7]

The chance of still having hot flushes and night sweats 12 months after starting HRT are 233 in 1000 women compared with 482 women in 1000 who took a placebo for 12 months. In other words, almost half of women aged 50 will naturally have fewer symptoms after 12 months but almost three-quarters will get relief if they take HRT. Figure 9.5 is based on extracts from a decision aid based on the evidence from the WHI study commissioned by the National Health and Medical Research Council (NHMRC), Australia.[8]

On the other hand, this same study showed that over 5 years a woman's risk of developing breast cancer increased from 11 in 1000 to 15 in 1000 on HRT, the chance of having an abnormal mammogram increased from 84 in 1000 to 139 in 1000, the risk of stroke increased from 4 in 1000 to 6 in 1000 and the risk of serious blood clots increased from 3 in 1000 to 8 in 1000.

Your probabilities need to be weighed up, together with what is most important to you. Decision aids for consumers, such as that

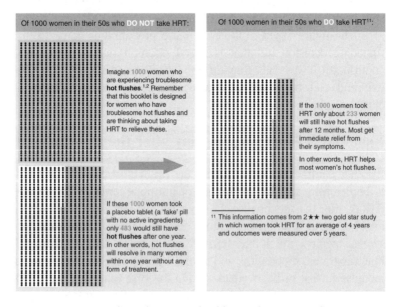

Figure 9.5 From *Making decisions: should I use hormone replacement therapy.*[8] (2 gold star evidence means a high quality randomised controlled trial)

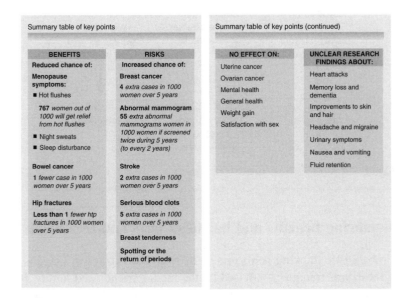

Figure 9.6 Balance sheet of risks and benefits of HRT treatment. From *Making decisions: should I use hormone replacement therapy?*[8]

from which the Figures have been reproduced, have been shown to help people become more actively involved in their healthcare decisions.[9] An example of a balance sheet or summary of these probabilities along with what we *don't* know about HRT is shown in Figure 9.6.

For other examples on the internet, see the patient decision aids designed by the Sydney Health Decision Group at www.health. usyd.edu.au/shdg and the Ottawa Health Research Institute http://decisionaid.ohri.ca/decaids.html.

Using probabilities to balance benefits and harms

The more we understand the probability that a test or treatment will cause a particular benefit or harm, the more informed our decision-making can be, as shown in Figure 9.7, and the more certain we can be of the results of our decisions.

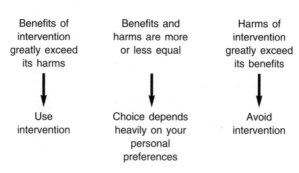

Figure 9.7 Weighing up benefits and harms

Balancing benefits and harms of tests and treatments

Probabilistic thinking helps protect us from the barrage of diagnostic tests and treatments advised by the media, friends and family. It also helps us to evaluate better the advice of our practitioners, whose concern about litigation may lead them to recommend unnecessary tests. Indeed, if we and our practitioners had more open discussions about the probable outcomes of different interventions, this might help reduce litigation.

> When people are led to expect a definite answer, a definite cure, they may quite understandably blame each other when things go wrong. The malpractice suit is the patient's way of blaming the doctor; the charge of 'non-compliance' is the doctor's way of blaming the patient. Under the Probabilistic Paradigm the fact that things may go wrong, and that it may or may not be anybody's fault, is acknowledged from the start.
>
> *Burstajn et al.*[10]

Practitioners should be judged on the process of care, rather than necessarily on the outcome of a disease or treatment. If a practitioner does the reasonable thing by declaring the risks and their probabilities based on the best available evidence and thereafter acts on this information, taking account of patient preferences, he or she has done the reasonable thing, regardless of the outcome.

Having information about probabilities allows us to decide if the dangers of a test or treatment outweigh their potential benefits. Ask your practitioner about probabilities; question how likely a good or bad health outcome might be. Think probabilistically when you read or hear health advice. By learning how to use probabilistic information, you will have an idea of what outcomes you can expect if you are ill and whether any interventions are likely to make a difference.

Summary

To estimate your chance of recovering from a disease, or of being helped or harmed by a test or treatment, you need probabilistic information. Taking a probabilistic approach to health issues is central to making better health decisions. This applies to the general public as well as your health practitioner. Probabilistic information:

- gives us an idea of the chance of a particular event occurring
- tells us what specific factors affect the probability of an event
- tells us whether an intervention changes the probability of an event.

Knowing the probabilities of the benefits and harms of different tests and treatments can help you and your practitioner make wise decisions that take account of your personal situation.

References

1. Doyle A. *The Sign of Four 1859–1930.*
2. Australian Institute of Health and Welfare. *Cancer in Australia 2001.* Canberra: AIHW, 2004.
3. Barratt A, Howard K, Irwig L, Salkeld G, Houssami N. Model of outcomes of screening mammography: information to support informed choices. *BMJ* 2005: doi:10.1136/bmj.38398.469479.8F.
4. Morris P, Leach A. Antibiotics for persistent nasal discharge (rhinosinusitis) in children. Cochrane Acute Respiratory Infections Group. *Cochrane Database of Systematic Reviews*, 2006:2.
5. McAlister D, Man-Son-Hing M, Straus S et al. Impact of a patient decision aid on care among patients with non-valvular atrial fibrillation: a cluster randomised trial. *Can Med Assn J* 2005;**173**:496–501.
6. *Making choices: treatments to prevent stroke in patients with atrial fibrillation.* http://www.canadianstrokenetwork.ca/eng/tools/index.php
7. Rossouw J, Anderson G, Prentice R et al. Risks and benefits of estrogen plus progestin in healthy postmenopausal women. *JAMA* 2002;**288**:321–33.
8. National Health and Medical Research Council. *Making Decisions: Should I use hormone replacement therapy?* Canberra, Australia: NHMRC, 2004: www.nhmrc.gov.au/publications/_files/wh37.pdf.
9. O'Connor A, Stacey D, Rovner D et al. Decision aids for people facing health treatment or screening decisions. *Cochrane Database of Systematic Reviews* 2003;2000(3).
10. Burstajn H, Feinbloom R, Hamm R, Brodsky A. *Medical Choices, Medical Chances.* New York: Routledge, 1990: 66.

IV

Evaluating the evidence

10

Judging which tests and treatments really work

Thinking straight about the world is a precious and difficult process that must be carefully nurtured.

Thomas Gilovich[1]

Whether sick or not, we are continuously offered health advice.

When we are sick, we are told that a new treatment will help us. When well, we are told how to avoid getting sick. Sometimes we're encouraged to have – or perhaps to avoid having – a screening test to detect disease early. Often we are warned that something causes cancer, heart disease, high blood pressure, and so on.

Some of this advice may be sound, but much is not. The important question is 'How do you tell which is which?' The answer is simple – ask if there is valid evidence to support the advice, irrespective of how competent or qualified the person giving you the advice seems to be. Competent practitioners should be prepared and willing to discuss the evidence supporting any advice that they offer.

The best way for you to decide whether the advice is good is to find out how good the supporting evidence is. The amount of effort that you put into this depends upon the importance of the decision. For minor issues you may not want to spend too much time, but, if it is an important decision for you, it will be well worth your while exploring the reliability of the evidence.

To do this, you need to find and make sense of the research literature on which the evidence is based. Don't be daunted. This is not nearly as complicated as it may sound, and doesn't require years of medical training. What it does require is the ability to distinguish between research that is well done and free of biases and research that is shaky and subject to biases and misinterpretation. This may sound difficult but is surprisingly straightforward if you follow some basic guides described in the following pages.

You can apply these guides to information in the media or on websites or to decisions made with your practitioner when you feel that the situation requires it. They can also be applied to articles in the medical literature, abstracts of which are available on the internet, as described in Chapter 15. Abstracts of studies are often structured with headings compatible with the following guides.

Is there an evidence-based practice guideline or systematic review of randomised trials?

As discussed in Part II, when you are examining the evidence about an intervention, the first question should always be: Is there an evidence-based practice guideline or systematic review of randomised trials? A guideline or systematic review based on the most recent, valid research, recommending how best to manage the disease or condition, is the single best source of evidence that you can get.

Be aware, however, that we are recommending *evidence-based* guidelines and reviews that come from the accumulated high-quality evidence from studies, and how to apply the evidence to individuals who vary in their preferences and characteristics. Not all practice guidelines are based on strong evidence. Some are just a consensus view of a group of experts without the search for impartial evidence. This is why you should establish whether a guideline is evidence based. Either ask your practitioner or read it yourself to determine whether it refers to up-to-date, valid research as its basis. Some guidelines are specifically written for consumers. Some summaries of systematic reviews are now available that have been written for the general public. Those that are not specifically intended for consumers may require your practitioner's help to interpret.

Remember, if a guideline or systematic review is evidence based:

- it will be recent, e.g. within the last 5 years; if it is not, ask if there is a more recent one.
- it will describe all the treatment options; systematic reviews should describe clearly what question they are addressing.
- it will describe outcomes that are person-centred (about quality of life and survival).
- it will describe both the benefits and harms of each option.
- it will describe how the best evidence was selected and report the highest level of evidence for each recommendation.

If there is no evidence-based guideline or systematic review on the health topic in question, you and your practitioner may need to make a decision based on existing studies on the disease and available tests or treatment options. We deal with a study's relevance first because, if it is not relevant to your situation, there is no point in assessing its quality.

Is the evidence relevant?

- The evidence should describe outcomes that are person-centred. They should tell you about survival or quality of life rather than surrogate measures such as laboratory results.
- The evidence should describe both harms and benefits and tell you how likely they are.
- The evidence should describe how tests and treatments compare with a wait and watch approach or each other.

Are the outcomes person-centred?

You need to make sure that a study that you are evaluating is relevant to your needs. It is important to know what the intervention's outcomes are, when they might occur, and how permanent and probable they might be. The evidence should demonstrate an effect on the length or quality of life rather than on some substitute intermediate endpoint. A study showing that drugs to dilate blood vessels (vasodilators) improve blood flow through the heart in people with heart failure is not, in itself, sufficient evidence for using the drugs. What would be relevant, however, is evidence that they help to reduce the symptoms and reduce the probability of requiring hospital treatment.

Are the harms described as well as the benefits?

You need to know about the chance of side effects and other downsides to treatments and tests, as well as when they might occur and if they are likely to be permanent. For example, chemotherapy for cancer may cause nausea, hair loss and weakness during the time it is taken. Another example is screening for early detection of disease. Screening may result in more people being recalled for further testing and invasive investigations than have the disease being screened for.

You also need to know the likelihood that you will benefit from treatment and tests. For example, as discussed in Chapter 9, the use of hormone therapy around the menopause may reduce symptoms of hot flushing and night sweats, but these benefits must be weighed up against its potential to increase the risk of breast cancer, blood clots, strokes and probably heart attacks.

Is the test or treatment compared with other suitable options?

Studies on new tests or treatments should show comparisons with the appropriate options – either a placebo or the best available existing treatments. Sometimes it will be important to know whether a test or treatment is better than doing nothing. But often there is already an effective treatment that is known to be superior to placebo. In such a situation we want evidence that the new intervention is going to have greater benefits and/or fewer harms than the existing one.

It has long been known, for example, that paracetamol offers effective long-term relief from the symptoms of osteoarthritis and has minimal side effects. On the other hand, non-steroidal anti-inflammatory drugs (NSAIDs) are associated with a high rate of gastrointestinal side effects. A systematic review of 15 randomised trials in the Cochrane Library showed that NSAIDs are more effective in reducing rest and movement-related pain in osteoarthritis, but the reduction in pain is small to modest (around 20 per cent).[2] As discussed earlier, if your level of pain is higher to start with, you will probably get a greater benefit from NSAIDs. However, NSAIDs are one and a half times more likely then paracetamol to give you gastric side effects such as nausea, indigestion and even bleeding. The review reports that 19 per cent of people on NSAIDs reported gastric side effects compared with 13 per cent on paracetamol. So neither treatment is risk free, but the chance of problems with NSAIDs is a little higher and this needs to be balanced against the amount of pain relief required. In view of the side effects of NSAIDs, it seems prudent to try paracetamol first and switch to NSAIDs only if pain relief is unsatisfactory.

Is the evidence reliable?

Reliability of evidence about an intervention, from the most to the least reliable, would go:

1. A systematic review of randomised controlled trials
2. A randomised controlled trial
3. Non-randomised studies:
   cohort studies and non-randomised trials
   population-based case–control studies
   hospital-based case–control studies
   other study types
4. Case reports and opinions.

Earlier in this book we introduced you to randomised controlled trials and systematic reviews, but this section will take you a bit further now that you know more about making sense of health advice.

Randomised controlled trials

We will start with an explanation of randomised controlled trials (RCTs) because it is easier to understand systematic reviews if you know something about RCTs first.

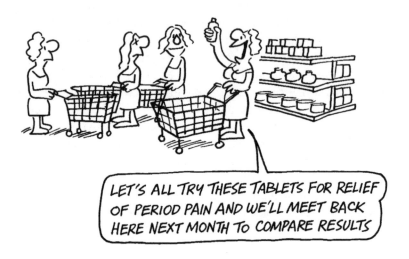

LET'S ALL TRY THESE TABLETS FOR RELIEF OF PERIOD PAIN AND WE'LL MEET BACK HERE NEXT MONTH TO COMPARE RESULTS

Unlike the scene in the cartoon, a good trial will:

- have a control group receiving the best existing treatment (or placebo, if there is no treatment)
- randomly allocate people to the intervention and control groups
- keep practitioners and study participants blind (or masked) to who is in which group
- follow up on everyone who was randomised to the various groups at the start of the trial.

This is the type of study that showed that an effective treatment for stomach ulcers is antibiotics and raised the alarm that antiarrhythmia drugs after a heart attack might have dangerous and previously unsuspected side effects. Randomised controlled trials also quashed the long-held theory that antioxidant vitamin tablets prevent cancer.[3]

Until RCTs showed otherwise, many doctors believed that the most effective way to treat early breast cancer was a mastectomy to remove all of the breast. They believed this because it was what they had been taught at medical school and it was what most specialists advised. This widely held belief has since been disproved by RCTs showing that women are just as likely to survive the cancer if they have less invasive surgery combined with radiotherapy.

Why 'controlled'?

As their name suggests, randomised controlled trials involve randomly allocating patients to either the active treatment or a comparison (control) group. This provides the all-important comparison. It is not much good knowing that a treatment leads to a 50 per cent recovery rate if you don't know how this compares with alternative treatments or even no treatment at all.

Similarly, if some people die while receiving a particular treatment, we don't know whether these deaths are a result of the treatment or the disease. But if there is another group not taking this treatment, a comparison of the two groups could help to establish whether the death rate is significantly higher in the group being treated.

Whether we can draw conclusions from comparing the outcomes of two groups depends on them being similar. If one group is sicker than the other, for example, this may bias the result of any comparison.

Why 'randomised'?

Randomly allocating patients to the comparison groups aims to reduce the chance of such biases occurring. It means that the groups start out with an equal chance of events occurring during the study, whether disease recurrence, side effects from treatment or symptom relief. In other words, it increases the likelihood that any differences in outcome between the groups are caused by the test or treatment and not other factors.

Sometimes randomisation is done as a cross-over trial. This means that people are first randomised to treatment A or B and then, after the outcome has been assessed, the groups cross over so that those who were receiving treatment A switch to treatment B and vice versa, and the outcomes are again measured. Of course, this type of trial can be done only if the outcomes are short and reversible – for example, to measure an intervention's effect on pain relief.

It is not enough to know that a treatment has been subjected to clinical trials. This means nothing more than that it has been tried. Clinical trials do not always include a control group and participants are not always randomly allocated. And controlled clinical trials may not be randomised. You really want to know that it is a randomised controlled trial.

The importance of 'blinding'

Blinding or masking is another important method for eliminating bias from RCTs when measuring the effects of an intervention. It aims to ensure that the researchers and participants do not know who is receiving treatment or placebo. This helps distinguish between real change resulting from the intervention and imagined change caused by the influence of enthusiasm and attention.

In an intervention study, the researchers and practitioners involved often have some prior expectation of the effect of the intervention being studied – otherwise, they probably would not be doing the study! These expectations may influence the way in which practitioners measure and record patients' responses, and can affect the validity of the results.

In the same way, participants often have some expectation of how the treatment will affect them, and might respond to the placebo effect. As well, when we are the target of special attention – as in being part of a trial – we tend to respond in a way that can affect our feeling of well-being. This phenomenon is sometimes referred to as the Hawthorne effect and can have a great impact on any therapy that we might be receiving.

To avoid these biases, ideally everyone involved in the trial – patients and practitioners (or researchers) – should be blinded to the treatment status. When the patients *and* the practitioners are blinded, this is referred to as a 'double-blinded' study.

If you are reviewing several RCTs on a particular intervention that show differing results, you should use blinding as a deciding factor. A study that is blinded or double-blinded is generally more reliable than the same type of study that is not.

If you want to know whether a study is an RCT and of good quality, check that the participants were randomised to the groups and that the participants and the practitioners were blinded. If these criteria are not declared, assume that they were not fulfilled.

Also check that all those randomised were followed up and included in the study results. Loss to follow-up is selection bias and may distort the comparison of the intervention and control arms.

Systematic reviews of randomised controlled trials

For a review to be systematic, the authors should declare whether they have:

* identified all the RCTs on the topic
* included all RCTs on the topic unless they do not meet the criteria for high-quality RCTs
* pooled the results into a large analysis, called a meta-analysis
* assessed whether there is variability in effects in different sorts of patients.

Even well-designed randomised trials can produce apparently differing results. The best method for evaluating such studies is through a systematic review, which examines the evidence from all of the good studies that have been done.

It was a systematic review, for instance, that finally accumulated enough evidence to persuade practitioners that there is value in chemotherapy for early breast cancer and antenatal steroids for infants born before term.

But be warned! Not all reviews are systematic reviews. Many reviews published in journals and elsewhere are no more than a collection of opinions that support a particular viewpoint.

The hazard of a haphazard review is obvious. Probably all of us are prejudiced and tend to focus on what we like to see. And, even worse, some of us tend to dismiss anything that does not suit our purpose. This makes it worthwhile to set certain rules before starting a review process. Reviews are scientific enquiries and they need a clear design to preclude bias.

A review that does not have a clear design to preclude bias is clearly not as reliable as a systematic review that, as its name suggests, takes a systematic approach to identifying the valid studies conducted on one topic and analysing the combined results.

Again, to determine whether a review is systematic, check whether the authors have declared that:

- all the RCTs on the topic have been identified
- all the RCTs have been included – unless they do not meet the criteria for high-quality RCTs
- the results have been pooled into a large analysis (meta-analysis).

The Cochrane Collaboration

The Cochrane Collaboration is an international movement of thousands of professionals and consumers who produce a regularly updated electronic library of the best available evidence about the effects of interventions. The Cochrane Library gives global access, to practitioners as well as consumers, to the most recent systematic reviews of RCTs on a rapidly expanding range of health topics. It contains thousands of systematic reviews of RCTs on a wide range of health treatment options. The abstracts or summaries of the reviews are available globally free of charge. In addition, some countries provide free access to the whole library: www.thecochranelibrary.com

The Cochrane Collaboration logo (opposite) illustrates a systematic review of data from seven RCTs. Each horizontal line represents the results of one trial (the shorter the line, the more certain the result) and the diamond represents their combined results. The vertical line indicates the position around which the horizontal lines would cluster if the two treatments compared in the trials had similar effects; if a horizontal line touches the vertical line, it means that that particular trial found no clear difference between the treatments. The position of the diamond to the left of the vertical line indicates that the treatment studied is beneficial.

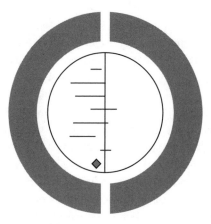

Figure 10.1 The Cochrane logo.

This diagram shows the results of a systematic review of RCTs of a short, inexpensive course of a corticosteroid given to women expected to give birth prematurely. The first of these RCTs was reported in 1972. The diagram summarises the evidence that would have been revealed had the available RCTs been reviewed systematically a decade later; it indicates strongly that corticosteroids reduce the risk of babies dying from the complications of immaturity. By 1991, seven more trials had been reported, and the picture in the logo had become still stronger. This treatment reduces the odds of the babies dying from the complications of immaturity by 30–50 per cent.

As no systematic review of these trials had been published until 1989, most obstetricians had not realised that the treatment was so effective. As a result, tens of thousands of premature babies have probably suffered and died unnecessarily (and cost healthcare services more than was necessary). This is just one of many examples of the human costs resulting from failure to perform systematic, up-to-date reviews of RCTs of health care.

Non-randomised studies

Cohort studies

Cohort studies are observational studies in which people are exposed to some factor of interest (for example, diet, smoking, occupation)

at the start of the study and then followed over a time period sufficient to allow any effects of that exposure to occur and be measured.
The important difference between a cohort study and a RCT is that,
in a cohort study, the groups are not randomised.

A good example of a cohort study is the Nurses Health Study,
coordinated by Harvard University in Boston, in which almost 100,000
nurses agreed to fill out questionnaires mailed to them annually asking
about their diet, health status, and so forth. Any reports of illnesses
were then confirmed by medical reports. This study provided information about the factors that may be involved in many diseases, including cancer, diabetes, osteoporosis and heart disease. It was also the
source of much of our earlier evidence that hormone replacement
therapy (HRT) reduced your chance of heart attack. As we have
mentioned a number of times in this book, when a randomised trial
was finally done, it proved the opposite in older women!

Case–control studies

Case–control studies are observational studies in which a group of
people who have a particular disease are observed to see whether
their past exposures to some factors differ from those of a similar
group who do not have the disease. They usually involve smaller
numbers of people. They can be either population based – all the
cases and controls are randomly selected from the same defined
geographical population – or hospital based – all the cases and
controls are selected from people attending a particular hospital. The
population-based case–control study yields stronger evidence than
one that is hospital based, which has many more sources of bias.

In case–control studies, information is usually obtained by
questioning the cases and controls. Naturally they will know
whether or not they have a certain disease, and this knowledge is
likely to influence the way in which they respond to questions,
which, in turn, can lead to recall bias – a type of measurement bias.

One important example of a population-based case–control
study investigated whether the risk of sudden infant death syndrome
(SIDS) is affected by a baby's sleeping position and the quantity of
bedding used. British researchers compared the situation of 72
infants who had died suddenly and unexpectedly (of whom 67 had

died from SIDS) with 144 control infants. They all were from a defined geographical area in the country – Avon and part of Somerset. The parents of the control infants were interviewed within 72 hours of the index infant's death. Information on all babies was collected on bedding, sleeping position, heating and recent signs of illness.[5]

Compared with the control infants, those who had died from SIDS were more likely to have been sleeping prone. As recall bias may occur in such a study (parents' reporting may be influenced by what they have heard about the disease), it is important for such results to be confirmed by RCTs or, at least, by cohort studies. The results of cohort studies have since confirmed that the prone sleeping position increases the risk of SIDS.[6] As it would not be ethical to randomise babies to different sleeping positions, a cohort study is likely to be the highest level of evidence available on this topic.

Cross-sectional analytical studies

Cross-sectional analytical studies are prone to more biases than cohort and case–control studies. These studies measure the two factors – exposure and disease – at the same time. For example, this method was used to see whether *herpes simplex* virus occurs more often in cervical cancer cells than in non-cancer cells. The problem with this approach is that it is unclear in which direction the causal arrow is pointing. We cannot tell from such a study whether the viruses cause cancer or whether the cancer cells are more susceptible to the growth of viruses.

Cross-sectional analytical studies are prone to selection bias. Consider what would happen if such a study were used to explore the relationship between cholesterol levels and the presence of coronary heart disease as measured by electrocardiography. There would be a problem in interpreting the results because, if high cholesterol does indeed cause a severe form of heart disease, by the time the study is ended and the sample population investigated, those with the highest levels of cholesterol are likely to have died from heart disease. In other words, this study will underestimate the relationship between high cholesterol levels and heart disease because it is based on a survivor population.

However, cross-sectional analytical studies are very useful for examining how well diagnostic tests identify the presence or absence of disease.

Opinions, case reports and anecdotes

Opinions, case reports and anecdotes all have one thing in common: they are largely based on personal experience that cannot be reliably generalised to other people. Their reliability as a source of evidence for an intervention is very weak except in highly specific situations that have to do with the nature of the illness being treated and the impact, immediacy and repeatability of the intervention's effect (see Chapter 8 on anecdotal evidence).

An example: judging whether you should switch to a Mediterranean diet rather than a low-fat diet if you are at higher risk of heart disease

Observational (non-randomised studies) across a number of countries have noted that people who have a so-called Mediterranean diet have a lower rate of heart attacks and strokes and live longer.[7,8] This seems plausible and, if you look for a randomised trial that tests this theory, you will find a recent one that randomly assigned people with higher than average risk of heart disease to either a low-fat diet or a Mediterranean diet. On first glance it looks like the Mediterranean diet was superior but there are some doubts raised when you look more closely.[9]

First, the researchers have mainly used surrogate outcome measures such as lipid levels and blood pressure. The additional benefits of a Mediterranean diet over and above a low-fat one were statistically significant but possibly wouldn't have much of an effect on clinical outcomes such as survival or heart attack rates. Also, they followed people for only 3 months so we don't know whether there was any effect on heart attack rates or survival.

Second, when you look more closely, the Mediterranean diet group got more educational material and free supplies of virgin olive oil and nuts, whereas the low-fat diet group did not have any education and did not get low-fat products supplied free of charge. You should be able to see the potential for bias here. You might decide to switch to a Mediterranean diet because you prefer the flavours and because it is unlikely to do you any harm. However, there is no conclusive evidence that it will reduce your chance of having a heart attack.

If you wish to test your skills on appraising health information, using what you've learnt in this chapter, try examples 1–4 in Chapter 15.

Summary

When trying to assess the effects of tests and treatments, we should look for valid evidence that is relevant to our needs. This may be provided in an evidence-based guideline or systematic review of randomised controlled trials.

To ensure that evidence about a test or treatment is relevant:

- The evidence should describe outcomes that are person centred. They should tell you about survival or quality of life rather than surrogate measures.
- The evidence should describe both harms and benefits and tell you how likely they are.

Studies vary in their reliability as a source of evidence. The following is the hierarchy of evidence about interventions, from strongest to weakest:

1. systematic reviews
2. randomised controlled trials
3. non-randomised studies
       cohort and other non-randomised trials
       population-based case–control studies
       hospital-based case–control studies
       other types of studies
4. opinions, case reports and anecdotes.

CHAPTER 10

References

1. Project PIaAL. Vital decisions: how Internet users decide what information to trust when they or their loved ones are sick: wwwintuteacuk/cgi-bin/redirpl?url=http://20721232103/pdfs/PIP_Vital_Decisions_May20 02pdf&handle=20028783. 2002.
2. Towheed T, Maxwell C, Judd M, Cath M, Hochberg M, Wells G. Acetaminophen for osteoarthritis. *Cochrane Database of Systematic Reviews.* 2006.
3. Bjelakovic G, Nikolova D, Simonetti R, Gluud C. Antioxidant supplements for preventing gastrointestinal cancers. *Cochrane Database of Systematic Reviews.* 2006.
4. Collaboration C. The Cochrane logo, available from: http://www.cochrane.org/logo/.
5. Fleming P, Gilbert R, Azaz Y. Interaction between bedding and sleeping position in the sudden infant death syndrome: a population based case-control study. *British Medical Journal* 1990;**301**:85–89.
6. Dwyer T, Ponsonby A, Newman, Gibbons. Prospective cohort study of prone sleeping position and sudden infant death syndrome. *The Lancet* 1991;**337**:1244.
7. Knoops K, de Groot L, Kronhout D, Perrin A-E, Moreiras-Varela O, Menotti A, et al. Mediterranean diet, lifestyle factors, and 10-year mortality in elderly European Men and Women. *JAMA* 2004;**292(12)**:1433–1439.
8. Trichopoulou A, Orfanos P, Morat T, Bueno-de-Mesquita B, et al. Modified Mediterranean diet and survival: EPIC-elderly prospective cohort study. *British Medical Journal* 2005;330:doi:10.1136/bmj.38415.8F.
9. Estruch R, Martinez-Gonzalez M, Corella D, Salas-Salvado J, Lopez-Sabater M, Vinyoles E, et al. Effects of a Mediterranean-Style Diet on Cardiovascular Risk factors: A Randomized Trial. *Annals of Internal Medicine* 2006;**145**:1–11.

11

What makes you sick?

A universe in which cause and effect always have a one to one correspondence with each other would be easier to understand, but it is obviously not the kind we inhabit.

Jerome Cornfield[1]

Living near power lines causes cancer. So does eating burnt steak. Stress at work will kill you. So might fluoridated water.

These are just some of the many recent claims about causes of disease. But how are these claims tested? We know that randomised controlled trials (RCTs) are best for testing the effect of interventions, but imagine randomly allocating people to live near powerlines so you could then measure the impact on cancer rates. Clearly, randomised controlled trials cannot be used in these situations.

So we have to look for other ways of assessing the influences of different exposures on health. 'Exposure' is the term used to describe a possible cause of disease such as something in our environment or a lifestyle behaviour. One way is to use randomised controlled trials to measure the impact of eliminating or reducing the exposure: measuring what happens to people's health when they quit smoking compared with people who keep on smoking.

Sometimes randomisation occurs 'naturally'. One study investigating the effects of wartime activity on combatants was naturally randomised because conscripts to the American army were selected by lottery on birth date. The findings showed an increased overall death rate, with much of the increase resulting from suicide and car accidents. The evidence from such a trial is stronger than from observational (non-randomised) studies.

When randomisation is impossible, observational studies can provide answers, based on observing what happens to people in various groups over a period of time while nature is allowed to take its course. Observational studies, such as cohort and case–control studies, differ from experimental studies in which some action is taken to change an outcome.

Observational studies are used:

- To investigate the causal link between an exposure or disease: for example, to follow a group of people to see whether those on a certain diet develop more heart disease or cancer than expected; or to observe mine workers over a time period to see whether they are at increased risk of lung disease.
- To follow up long-term rare effects: for example, a medication that has been approved on the grounds of an RCT showing

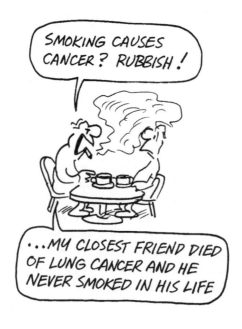

short-term benefits can be followed up to assess its long-term outcomes by an observational study.

• To calculate risk predictors of disease: for example, to establish whether age, family history of breast cancer and the number of births are predictors of breast cancer risks.

How to know when a relationship is causal?

Even when there is an association between two factors – such as using a walking stick and grey hair, or eating carrots and car accidents – the one does not necessarily cause the other. To determine whether a condition or disease is actually caused by something we do or eat requires that several criteria are present.

Does X cause Y?

1. The evidence about the relationship should be from a reliable source – the best possible study type.
2. The exposure to the supposed cause should occur before the outcome.
3. There should be a strong relationship between the supposed cause and the outcome.
4. There should be a dose–response or exposure–response relationship between the supposed cause and outcome, that is, the greater the exposure, the more likely someone is to get a disease.
5. There should not be any other factor that could explain the relationship.
6. The same results should be shown in several studies.
7. The relationship should make sense.

Is evidence about the relationship from a reliable source?

In other words, how good is the quality of the studies providing the evidence? The quality of evidence from various study types is given in Chapter 10. Obviously we can rely more on an RCT than on evidence from observational (non-randomised) studies. For example, an RCT showing that lowering blood pressure in people with high blood pressure will reduce the risk of stroke is better evidence that high blood pressure causes strokes than a cohort study suggesting an association between high blood pressure and stroke. Cohort and population-based case–control studies would provide better evidence than hospital-based case–control studies.

Did exposure to the supposed cause occur before the outcome?

This is about the causal arrow. Obviously studies showing that the supposed cause is present before the outcome provide stronger evidence. For example, a cross-sectional analytical study showing that people who have had a heart attack are more likely to exercise does not constitute strong evidence that exercise causes heart attacks. It just means that there is an association between exercise and heart attacks. We can't tell which one led to the other because the cross-sectional study design is like a 'snapshot' at a certain point and doesn't tell you anything about the sequence of events over time. It is quite possible that people who had heart attacks started exercising because of it and that accounts for the association.

Is there a strong relationship between the supposed cause and the outcome?

If an observational study shows that smokers are nine times more likely to develop lung cancer than non-smokers, this is a strong relationship and is likely to be causal and not the result of biases in the study. But if a study shows that people with a certain exposure are 1.3 times more likely to develop a certain disease, this is not a strong finding and may well be explained by some bias in the study design and not reflect a causal relationship.

Is there a dose–response or exposure–response relationship between the supposed cause and the outcome?

The evidence for causality is stronger if it can be shown that, the higher the dose or the longer the time of exposure, the greater the risk of the disease. For example, the risk of lung cancer increases progressively as the number of cigarettes smoked each day increases. In Chapter 12 we mention the dose–response relationship in the example about the relationship between fruit juice consumption and Alzheimer's disease.

Can the relationship be explained by anything else?

Even in well-designed studies, there might be important differences at the outset between the groups being compared. Supposing a study is planned to find out if workers in a particular industry have a higher risk of developing lung cancer than the general population. There is already good evidence that smoking causes lung cancer so, if the workers in this particular industry happen to be heavier smokers than the population with which they are being compared, it would not be surprising if the study showed an increased incidence of lung cancer in that industry. The question is: can this increase in lung cancer be attributed to the working environment or is it the result of other factors? In this example smoking is a confounder, which may bias the results. But unlike many biases, confounders can be adjusted for in the analysis. Age is a very common confounder because disease rates are usually closely related to age. Consequently, differences in age between the 'exposed' and 'non-exposed groups' might well be the cause of any differences between them in disease occurrence.

Always check whether studies have identified and taken account of potential confounders that may influence the comparison. They can do this by showing that the potential confounders occur equally across all groups, or by using some statistical techniques to adjust for them. If the study does not state that potential confounding factors have been adjusted or controlled for, assume that it has not been done.

Are the same results shown in several studies?

The more studies that show the same sort of effect, the more confident you can be in the evidence. Just as there are systematic reviews of RCTs on the effects of interventions, so too there are systematic reviews of observational studies on the causes of diseases. Similarly, we need to be sure that all the high-quality studies have been identified and used.

Does the relationship make sense?

The fact that some process seems to make sense is not, in itself, good evidence. It does, however, add weight if the criteria described above have been fulfilled. When an outcome is expected based on an understanding of biological mechanisms, this has more credibility than something that is contrary to biological expectations. We know, for example, that cigarette smoke reaches the lung, so information about a link between smoking and lung cancer is more believable than, say, suggesting a relationship between loud music and lung cancer. If you want to test your skill in assessing a causal relationship, turn to example 5 in Chapter 15.

Summary

When it is impossible to randomise people to study the cause or a predictor of disease, observational studies can provide useful information about the following:

- Whether exposure to some environment or behaviour causes a disease; for example, to see whether diet has an effect on heart disease or cancers; or whether certain occupations cause specific diseases.
- To follow up long-term rare effects; for example, to assess long-term outcomes of medication that has been approved on the grounds of an RCT showing its short-term benefits.
- For calculating risk predictors of disease; for example, to see whether the risk of breast cancer can be

continued

predicted by factors such as age, family history of breast cancer and number of births.

Criteria to help you determine whether a relationship is causal include:

* The evidence comes from a reliable source.
* The exposure to the supposed cause occurred before the outcome.
* The relationship between supposed cause and outcome is strong.
* There is a dose–response or exposure–response relationship between the supposed cause and outcome.
* The relationship cannot be explained by any other factors.
* Other studies show the same results.
* The relationship makes sense.

Reference

1. Cornfield J, Haenszel W, Cuyler Hammond E. Smoking and lung cancer: recent evidence and a discussion of some questions. *J Natl Cancer Inst* 1959;**22**:173–203.

V

Improving your healthcare

12

Finding the best evidence

Knowledge is not power. Getting the right information and learning how to apply it to your life is power.

Powter[1]

When you're looking for information to help guide your health decisions, there are a few important criteria to consider. Your decision should be based on the best available research evidence, and it is more likely to be meaningful if it can be personalised in some way so that it helps you to consider what's important to you.

This was the conclusion of a systematic review of randomised trials about effective ways to communicate with patients. The review found that there are many useful formats. But no matter what format the information comes in – whether verbally or in a magazine article or from an interactive website – you should remember these criteria.[2] And, ideally, the information should be able to answer all five of our 'smart health choice' essential questions.

Read on and you will discover some practical tips for finding and assessing the best evidence, whether from a practitioner, the Cochrane Library, the internet, organisations, universities, libraries or companies.

Evidence from your practitioner

Verbal

It is often enough to have your practitioner discuss with you what the evidence-based guidelines recommend, or tell you about recent systematic reviews or randomised controlled trials. Whether this will be sufficient will depend on the seriousness of your condition and your relationship with the practitioner. Don't forget to ask about the evidence, even if it is not offered. Asking the question 'What's the evidence?' is more likely to obtain a detailed response than simply asking 'Is there good evidence to support this?' Some cancer specialists are realising that it is sometimes difficult to absorb every-thing that is being discussed and they offer to record the consulta-tion so that cancer patients can go over things and think about them at home.

Written leaflets, booklets

It is often useful to have some written information to take away to consider and discuss with others. It may be some information prepared for patients and consumers, or evidence-based guidelines or even systematic reviews or randomised controlled trials.

However, not all written information is evidence based or of good quality. An audit of breast screening invitation letters across seven countries showed that they tended to over-emphasise the benefits of mammography and under-emphasise potential risks. In most cases, women were not given detailed information about the likely impact of mammography screening.[3]

A very useful checklist has been developed called the DISCERN instrument. It can be downloaded free or used online at www.discern.org.uk and is designed to help assess the quality of consumer health information. If you really want to check out the reliability of a source when trying to answer the 'smart health choice essential' questions, then the DISCERN instrument is excellent.[4] The main quality criteria are as shown in the box.

DISCERN

Section 1: Is the publication reliable?

1. Are the aims clear?
2. Does it achieve its aims?
3. Is it relevant?
4. Is it clear what other sources of information were used to compile the publication?
5. Is it clear when the information used or reported in the publication was produced?
6. Is it balanced and unbiased?
7. Does it provide details of additional sources of support and information?
8. Does it refer to areas of uncertainty?

Section 2: How good is the quality of information on treatment choices?

9. Does it describe how each treatment works?
10. Does it describe the benefits of each treatment?
11. Does it describe the risks of each treatment?
12. Does it describe what would happen if no treatment were used?
13. Does it describe how the treatment choices affect overall quality of life?
14. Is it clear that there may be more than one possible treatment choice?
15. Does it provide support for shared decision-making?

Section 3: Overall rating of the publication

16. Based on the answers to all of the above questions, rate the overall quality of the publication as a source of information about treatment choices

Electronic

Increasingly, this is the way practitioners will be accessing information for you. Keeping written materials up to date is becoming impossible in this rapidly changing world. Rather than digging out a photocopied leaflet from the bottom of the filing cabinet when you present with a whiplash injury, practitioners will be more likely to download the most recent consumer version of evidence-based guidelines and print you a copy to take home, complete with instructions on neck exercises and evidence-based advice on what to do and what not to do. These resources are often available in several languages. Another good example is *Cervical Screening: the facts*, available in 19 languages at http://www.cancerscreening.nhs.uk/index.html

Practitioners may also search the medical literature for you if there is time during the consultation. You can even follow up on these sources at home. As we have mentioned already, the Cochrane Library is available free in a number of countries and Medline, which is run by the US National Library of Medicine, is available all over the world via PubMed. A more comprehensive list of resources is available in Chapter 15.

Instead of thumbing through a vaccine handbook when asked what vaccines you will need for an upcoming backpacking trip to south-east Asia, practitioners may look up the Centers for Disease Control and Prevention website at www.cdc.gov/travel. This website is updated daily and gives advice about the latest outbreaks around the world including bird flu and, before that, SARS (severe acute respiratory syndrome). You can type in what countries and regions you will be visiting and get advice on immunisations and antimalarials, plus other valuable information about water quality and other travel hazards.

Below is an example of how you might obtain evidence from a practitioner. In brackets we show how the conversation relates to the five questions raised in Chapter 5.

Robert is travelling back from a trip to the USA, browsing through a magazine he had bought there. He notices an advertisement for a particular antibiotic to treat childhood ear infections, which describes what antibiotics are and how they work, but does not provide any information on whether they **do** actually work. Robert ponders on this. A while back, his 3-year-old son, Jeremy, had a rash that was thought to be a side effect of a course of antibiotics. This has made Robert well aware that any potential benefit may be bought at some harm.

A few weeks later, Jeremy develops a fever and complains of a sore ear, and Robert takes him to his doctor, Frank, who diagnoses a middle-ear infection.

Frank: 'A course of antibiotics should do the trick. Keeping in mind that he reacted adversely to the last lot, I'll prescribe a different one this time.'

Robert: 'I was wondering, Frank, are antibiotics really necessary? I'm loath to give him yet another course unless it's absolutely necessary. What will happen if we wait for a while to see if it gets better?' [Q1: What will happen if I wait and watch?]

Frank: 'Ear infections are likely to be bacterial, and I always prescribe antibiotics in these situations.'

Robert: 'I see. So are antibiotics the only option then?' [Q2: What are my options?]

Frank: 'Well another option is to treat with paracetamol to relieve the fever and pain, but it won't have any effect on the infection itself or possible complications from the infection. Remember, Robert, even though antibiotics have risks, they're very low.'

Robert: 'Mmmm. I suppose what I'm after is some idea of how effective antibiotics really are for ear infections. You say the risk is low, but it may not be worth taking if there's no proven benefit. And I know paracetamol is pretty safe.' [Q3: What are the benefits and harms of the options?] 'Is there an evidence-based guideline? Or a randomised controlled trial?'

Frank: 'As a matter of fact, I've used the Cochrane Library a number of times. Let's see what it says about ear infections.'

Turning to the computer on his desk, Frank searches for the relevant abstract and finds a systematic review of several randomised controlled trials.[5] To his surprise, antibiotics do not seem to have any effect in reducing pain during the first day of the infection. After an average of 4 days, 80 per cent of patients settle without treatment. However, for those 20 per cent of children who still have pain after that time, antibiotics do seem to help.

Frank: 'Well, there you are then. From this it would seem there's no harm in waiting for 24 hours to see how Jeremy settles just with paracetamol – if that's what you want to do. I'll give you a prescription for antibiotics just in case you need it after that.' [Q4: How do the benefits and harms weigh up for me?]

Robert: 'Sounds perfect, thank you. I'll let you know how he does. By the way, I found that very helpful. I have all the information I need for now. Thanks again.' [Q5: Do I have enough information to make a choice?]

This is a very satisfactory outcome for Robert and Jeremy, and for Frank too.

Evidence from companies providing products and services

Companies – whether they are making pharmaceuticals, vitamins or diagnostic tests – generally have one major aim: to make profits, whether for their shareholders or private owners. It is important to keep this in mind when evaluating claims made by those with a commercial interest at stake – especially if they are superlative claims substantiated by poor evidence based on inconclusive studies or theoretical explanations of how the product SHOULD work!

Many drug companies have websites with substantial information about their products. You will recall the warnings earlier in this book about being aware of some of the pitfalls of taking evidence at face value where there are commercial interests at stake.

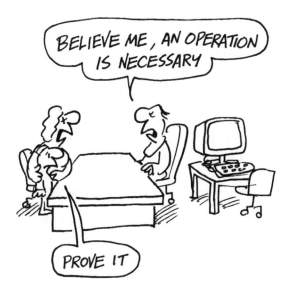

Ask to see the evidence for their claims. And evaluate it using the same criteria that you would use for assessing any research (see validity guides in Chapter 9). Using these criteria will help you determine if the research has been designed to push a particular interest.

Evidence from organisations

Many organisations provide health information. You may find yourself looking up information and it can be difficult to tell what's reliable and what's not. Try to answer the five 'smart health choice' questions and keep in mind the DISCERN criteria when you are trying to assess how reliable a source is. Websites for the following categories are listed in the section on Useful contacts later in the book.

Evidence from the Cochrane Library

As discussed in Chapter 10, the Cochrane Library provides what is almost certainly the most powerful, growing, single source of evidence about the effects of healthcare. It provides regularly updated, electronically accessible systematic reviews on thousands of treatments. Recently the Cochrane Collaboration decided to withdraw any systematic review that had not been updated within the last 5 years. So you should be fairly confident that the information there is up to date. Another new initiative is that many of the systematic reviews now have lay summaries in plain English, which should make the evidence much more accessible to everyone, not just high-powered researchers!

Consumer health bodies and self-help groups

There are many groups that have been largely set up by consumers to support each other and offer information, advice and advocacy for others suffering with the same condition. One example in the UK is Breast Cancer Care (www.breastcancer.org.uk) and in Australia the National Breast Cancer Network of Australia (www.bcna.org.au) whose website contains a range of patient stories, brochures, booklets and links to other organisations. Newsletters and support groups are also linked. A more comprehensive list is included at the back of this book.

General government health departments and other official organisations

These can provide information about health policies and contact details for other organisations. Some may be able to provide information about hospitals and other health services, such as whether they are accredited or have services for patient support or complaints. They may also be able to investigate if you have had problems with a health service or product. In the UK the NHS National Library for Health at http://www.library.nhs.uk/ provides evidence-based guidelines and consumer information. In Australia, the National Health and Medical Research Council (NHMRC) produces a variety of information booklets and guidelines aimed at consumers and health professionals (www.nhmrc.gov.au/publications). State governments also provide consumer health information on their websites.

Cancer councils and specialist associations

Cancer councils are generally community-based organisations committed to preventing cancer and enhancing the quality of life for people with cancer and their families. They provide information, education and support, and also fund research and professional development. For the UK go to Cancer Research UK (www.cancer researchuk.gov) and in Australia links to the Cancer Council in each state can be found at Cancer Council Australia (www.cancer.org.au/ Home.html). Specialist associations exist for many diseases, disorders and other conditions. To find a specialist service or a medical specialist appropriate to your needs in your area, in the UK look via NHS Direct (www.nhsdirect.nhs.uk/). In Australia the Australian Medical Directory, apart from listing the details of all registered medical practitioners, includes a section on professional and specialist medical groups.

Complementary medicine or alternative health associations

There are many complementary medical associations, representing both medically qualified and non-medical practitioners. Although there is some good quality research in this area, on the whole there are fewer high-quality studies investigating complementary than orthodox therapies. The same evaluation criteria should be applied to all doctrines of healthcare. Examples of good studies on complementary medicine are available on the Cochrane Collaboration website and are published in major medical journals.

University research groups

Some research groups make their evidence-based tools available for consumers on their own websites. Decision aids, such as the ones we saw earlier for preventing strokes in patients with atrial fibrillation, can be found on the Ottawa Health Research Institute website (decisionaid.ohri.ca/decaids.html) and the Sydney Health Decision Group website (www.health.usyd.edu.au/shdg). The German

Institute for Quality and Efficiency in Healthcare has been publishing consumer-friendly versions of Cochrane reviews at Informed Health Online, www.informedhealthonline.com. Harvard University also has a disease risk assessment tool at www.your diseaserisk.harvard.edu, and the list goes on.

Local hospitals and family practices

Some local hospitals may have information resources or ideas on where to get the information that you need. Increasingly, the larger hospitals in many countries will provide substantial patient information on their websites. For example, Great Ormond Street Hospital for Children in London (UK) and the Royal Children's Hospital in Melbourne (Australia) have comprehensive sections for parents and children (www.ich.ucl.ac.uk and www.rch.org.au). Increasingly, many general practices are putting up websites with information about their doctors and practice facilities. Some are also adding recommended health information websites.

Surfing the internet yourself

Doing research on the Web is like using a library assembled piece-meal by pack rats and vandalized nightly.

Roger Ebert

Information is the currency of democracy.

Thomas Jefferson

Media manipulation in the U.S. today is more efficient than it was in Nazi Germany, because here we have the pretense that we are getting all the information we want. That misconception prevents people from even looking for the truth.

Mark Crispin Miller

The twenty-first century is a time in history like no other when one considers the amount of information available to the average person each day through radio, TV and the internet. An estimated 13.9 million households (57 per cent) in the UK had home internet access in April 2006, with similar figures for other developed countries such as Australia, Canada and the USA. Each year, this proportion increases and over half of these households now have broadband connections, enabling linkage to larger quantities of information at higher speed.

Just from the brief list of organisations and sources that we have shown above, you might already be starting to feel overwhelmed. The problem of information overload is only going to get worse as more and more people publish information on the web.

But be aware that much is unreliable; it can take quite a bit of time and effort to determine what is valid and relevant to your needs. It would probably be unwise to make major decisions about your healthcare solely on the basis of information obtained through the internet, without first discussing it with your practitioner and checking the quality of its source as described earlier in this book.

One way of increasing the chance of getting valid guidelines or other high-quality research is to restrict your searches to university or government agencies. You can do this in some search engines. For example, Google Scholar (www.scholar.google.com) searches academic publications, professional organisations, universities and peer-reviewed papers.

This problem of information overload has been recognised and many governments are establishing consumer information portals. The UK has the National Electronic Library for Health www.library. nhs.uk/Default.aspx and the Australian Government's one is called Health Insite www.healthinsite.gov.au. You can be fairly confident in the reliability of information on these sites because they have been checked by an expert in advance. You still need to be alert, however, because bad information can still slip through the net.

How people use the internet in healthcare decision-making

The internet is a common source of health information for consumers. Surveys of internet use have consistently shown that more than half of internet users access health information. US reports claim that 62 per cent of internet users, or 73 million people, in the USA have gone online at some point in search of health information and about 6 million people go online for advice in a typical day.[6,7] Most commonly people were looking for disease information, material about weight loss and facts about prescription drugs. Typical health advice seekers went online only occasionally to look up something specific and most of them did so without getting *any* advice from family, practitioners or others on *where* to look for reliable information. Despite this lack of guidance, most people said that they found useful websites and that it had helped them in their health-care decision-making.

People varied a lot in whether they would systematically check that a site could be trusted. Only a quarter said that they always looked for quality criteria such as the source of the information and when it was posted. But most people (73 per cent) said that at some point they had decided not to rely on a particular website. Most commonly they had rejected it because it appeared to be overly commercial, they couldn't work out how up to date it was, it had an unprofessional design or they couldn't find the source of the information.

There's no doubt that with so many home computers now linked to the internet 'surfing the net' is a very convenient way for patients to look things up. No longer do you have to go to your local library or bookstore in search of the information that you want. The internet is not just convenient, it's also flexible. People generally don't know in advance how much health information they will need. At different points in time they will want different information on different topics and on the same topics at different levels of detail. The internet can accommodate this constantly changing requirement for information.

One UK study of cancer patients and their families found that people used the internet in many different ways. Some of the questions for which they sought answers were very similar to the five questions from the 'smart health choice essentials'. They fit under seven broad categories suggested by Ziebland and quoted here below:[8]

1. *Before visiting the doctor*: to discover the possible meaning of symptoms.

2. *During investigations*: to seek reassurance that the doctor is doing the right tests; to prepare for the results; and to improve the value of the consultation.

3. *After the diagnosis*: to gather information about the cancer (including information that is 'difficult' to ask about directly); to seek advice about how to tell children; to contact online support groups; to seek second opinions; to make sense of the stages of disease; to interpret what health professionals have said; and to tackle isolation.

4. *When choosing treatments*: to find information about treatment options and side effects, experimental treatments, research, and alternative and complementary treatments.

5. *Before treatment*: to find out what to take to hospital, what will happen, what it will be like, what to expect of recovery, how to identify and prepare questions to ask the doctors.

6. *Short-term follow-up*: to find information about side effects, reassurance about symptoms, advice about diet, complementary treatments, benefits and finances; to check that the treatment was optimal and what the perceived therapeutic benefits are.

7. *Long-term follow-up*: to share experience and advice, contact support groups and chat rooms, campaign about the condition, make anonymous enquiries.

The relationship between the internet and the health practitioner

Clearly, there's no getting past the convenience and flexibility of the internet for people to access health information and this is likely to become even more commonplace. There's no delay or wait for an appointment to start seeking answers to health-related questions. And people are using 'the net' for this and other aspects of their lives. In a similar way, we no longer need to pay our bills in person or even by post; we can do our banking online and even book our holidays without going anywhere near a travel agent.

What, then, is the role of the health practitioner in this age of 'armchair information'? Despite accessing web-based information from home, most people *still* prefer to get definitive advice from their health practitioner. But they would like to supplement it with other resources and would appreciate their doctor pointing them towards reliable internet resources. The consultation of the future is likely to take on a very different shape as a result of this. Practitioners will increasingly suggest to patients that they refer to particular resources and consider their options before returning to discuss further. This gives people time to reflect on good quality information and discuss it with their family and friends if desired. As practitioners increasingly practise evidence-based healthcare the involvement of patients in the decision-making process becomes much more of a partnership, and guiding patients towards good quality information sources is an important part of their role.

Looking for good quality health information on the internet

The UK Department of Health has stressed the importance of access to good quality information in the White Paper *Better Information, Better Choices, Better Health – Putting information at the centre of health* (December 2004).

Over the past decade several tools have been developed to try to rate the quality of health information on websites, but most of them have not been very useful and have been discontinued. Recently, the British Medical Association (BMA) has suggested that there are six broad issues that should be considered when looking at a health information website. A similar list has been developed by the Australian Government's Health Insite and the US National Institutes for Health.

BMA quality criteria for health websites (www.bma.org.uk)

1. Is the site regularly updated? Information on the review process – for example, the most recent review date – should be given on the site.
2. Does the site give references and sources for the information it provides?
3. Does the site provide information about who compiled the site (the organisation or individual)?

4. Does the organisation give an address/other contact details?
5. Spelling and grammatical mistakes – more than a couple of these indicate a weak site that has not been properly edited or reviewed.
6. Is the organisation trying to sell something? If so, be wary of the information.

Government websites for reliable health information

A number of government initiatives have been set up to provide consumers with good quality health information. In the UK, the National Library for Health has several patient resources that are reliable and useful: www.library.nhs.uk/forpatients

1. NHS Direct has been established to provide 24-hour e-health and telephone support to consumers to enable them to make decisions about their healthcare and that of their families. It includes a health encyclopaedia, answers to common health questions, self-help guides, a health magazine, enquiry facilities and information about finding a health service.
2. Best Treatments (produced by BMJ Publishers and free to UK residents), contains plain language summaries of randomised controlled trials and systematic reviews of treatments.
3. DiPEx is a database of patient experiences that we discuss further in Chapter 13.
4. Patient.co.uk contains free health information for common general practice problems.

The US National Library of Medicine has an extensive database of good quality information about over 700 diseases and conditions. Medline Plus (http://medlineplus.gov) also includes help with searching the internet for health information and lists of hospitals and physicians in the USA. It has extensive information about prescription and non-prescription drugs, health information from the media and also links to clinical trials.

The Australian Government has established Health Insite (www.healthinsite.gov.au) a consumer health information website that includes only content that meets certain assessment criteria and standards.

Media reports

The media are an ever-present and powerful source of health information for us in today's world. In earlier chapters we highlighted the fact that many media stories rely heavily on the power of the anecdote and the telling of one person's story. These stories can often be very helpful in providing insight into the experience of particular illnesses. As with any information source, there are good and bad examples. There are well-researched and carefully prepared reports, and there are the sensational and often misleading headlines in the tabloid newspapers.

Some evidence-based practitioners have been sharing their expertise with journalists via training workshops in recent years to help improve the accuracy of reporting on health news items. As well, several initiatives have been set up to give the media and its audiences some feedback about the accuracy of media reports and the reliability of the research they are covering. These include Media Doctor Australia (www.mediadoctor.org.au/) and Media Doctor Canada (http://www.mediadoctor.ca), while Health News Review performs a similar function in the United States (http://www.health newsreview.org). In the UK, the Hitting the Headlines service (http://www.york.ac.uk/inst/crd/hth.htm) provides a rapid analysis of media reports about research. Looking at the stories featured on these web services makes it clear that there is great variability in the quality of media reporting. You certainly shouldn't be relying purely on what the headlines say when making important health decisions.

Making sense of health stories in the media

Medical breakthroughs make great headlines. Each week, news outlets report on research published in journals or promoted by researchers, companies or other agencies. However, these headlines should not be taken at face value. The consistent message of this book is that you should always question the level of evidence that lies behind the catchy headlines.

Here's a good example. In October 2006, the *American Journal of Medicine* published a study that reported an association between regular fruit juice consumption and a reduced chance of developing Alzheimer's disease. Headlines read 'Drinking juice may slash Alzheimer's risk', 'Drinking juice might stall Alzheimer's' and 'Juices may cut Alzheimer's risk', claiming that the study had produced 'powerful results' that 'the risk was 76 per cent lower for those who drank juice more then three times a week compared with those who drank it less than once a week'.

However, what is not explained by the media is that this study was a cohort design and, as discussed earlier in this book, such a design is prone to bias. It may be that people who drink juice more than three times per week are in better health generally, exercise more, and have higher education levels and better diets. What we would really need to do to answer this question is randomise people to high and lower fruit juice consumption for a period of perhaps 10 years (as this was the timeframe for the other study). It may be that we find through this process that increased fruit juice consumption actually has the opposite effect and increases the chance of Alzheimer's disease.

Apart from study design it is important to look at the actual (or absolute) numbers of people affected by a treatment or behaviour change. When the original article is considered, there is a very strange pattern in the results. The number of people probably free of Alzheimer's disease is *greater* in people who drink *juice less than weekly* (compared with once or twice a week). The number free of Alzheimer's disease drops to 16 per 100 with one to two juices per week and then increases to 49 per 100 with three or more juices per week. It is very difficult to explain why the Alzheimer's disease risk doesn't consistently fall with greater juice consumption. This is called a dose–response relationship and is another thing to consider when looking for a cause-and-effect relationship.

A similar example comes from a media report that 'decaffeinated coffee may cause heart problems'. When you look more closely at this story, the study was not a randomised trial and was prone to bias. You may want to change from drinking decaffeinated coffee to the standard variety, but it should not be done on the basis of changing your heart disease risk.

As we are bombarded with new health headlines in the media each day, it can be difficult to know how to make sense of them all. There are two common pitfalls in media reporting of research. One is that they overstate the validity of results from studies that are not randomised controlled trials and therefore prone to bias. Second, they often report effects in relative terms rather than absolute. A 20 per cent reduction in something that is very common will have a greater impact than a 20 per cent reduction in a rare event. For example, if a disease is fairly common (for example, the common cold) you might estimate that 80 out of 100 people in the community will get one over winter. A treatment that reduces your chance of getting the common cold by 20 per cent will mean that only 64 people out of 100 will get 'a cold' if they all take the treatment. On the other hand, if the treatment is less common (for example, for heart attacks) we might estimate that 5 out of 100 people might have a heart attack over the next 10 years. If a treatment reduces the chance of having a heart attack by 20 per cent then only 4 people out of 100 will have one.

For heavy duty research

University and other libraries and Medline, an electronic database of the medical literature, provide useful sources if you want to explore a health issue in great depth.

Medline, which is now available free on the web, provides a database of the titles and abstracts of articles in the most important medical journals. Once you have located a study that looks relevant, you can follow it up from the reference provided. Articles are indexed by the subject that they cover – such as 'breast neoplasms' – as well as methodological headings – such as 'randomised controlled trial'.

You don't necessarily need to be a student or staff member to gain access to a university library. In many countries they are available for use by the general public, and it may be worth checking out your local institutions' policies. They can be useful for providing access to electronic databases, such as Medline, or to hard copy journals.

When searching journals, remember that the most reliable ones are those that are subject to quality control by peer review. This means that, before an article is published, it is submitted to other experts in the area of interest for their comments. To establish whether a journal is peer reviewed look in the 'instructions to authors' section where the peer review process is usually described. Examples of some such high quality journals include, *The Lancet, New England Journal of Medicine, British Medical Journal, Journal of the American Medical Association* and *Annals of Internal Medicine.* Many of these are also available on the internet.

Other libraries that can be useful are: local libraries, which can have links to other, larger libraries; state libraries; and libraries of specialist associations.

Summary

Evidence can be obtained from a variety of sources.

- **From your practitioner:** ask your practitioner about evidence-based guidelines, recent systematic reviews or randomised controlled trials. You may also want to take written copies of these home. You or your practitioner may also have access to electronically accessible databases that should provide these sources of evidence. Health practitioners can be a helpful source to guide patients towards reliable information.
- **From companies providing products and services:** the aim of companies is usually to make profits. Keep this in mind, especially if the claims are based on poor

continued

or inconclusive studies or theoretical explanations. Companies making claims should be able to provide the evidence to support them.

- **From other organisations:** consumer-friendly information can also be obtained from health departments, cancer councils and other associations dealing with particular diseases.
- **From the internet:** although plentiful, much information from the internet is unreliable. It would be wise to discuss any information with your practitioner and appraise its quality. Certain factors should be considered (at a minimum) when finding reliable internet information:
  - who compiled the site and are they likely to have any conflict of interest?
  - how up to date is the site?
  - what is the source of its information?
  - government-funded consumer websites tend to have explicit quality assurance processes and are likely to be quite reliable.
- **From the media**: be cautious about media stories and headlines that make bold or sensational claims. Remember to ask yourself about the likelihood of benefits and harms from a test or treatment. Media headlines about health discoveries should be tested by looking into the study design and consider whether effects are reported in absolute (actual) numbers.
- **For heavy duty research:** university and other libraries and Medline, an electronic database of the medical literature, provide useful sources if you want to explore a health issue in great depth.

References

1. Powter S. *Stop the Insanity*. Australia: Orion, 1994.
2. Trevena L, Davey H, Barratt A, Butow P, Caldwell P. A systematic review on communicating with patients about evidence. *J Eval Clin Pract* 2006;**12**(1):13–23.
3. Jorgensen K, Gotzsche P. Content of invitations for publicly funded screening mammography. *BMJ* 2006;**332**:538–41.
4. Charnock D, Sheppard S. DISCERN Instrument: www.discern.org.uk, 2006.
5. Glasziou P, Del Mar C, Sanders S, Hayem M. Antibiotics for acute otitis media in children. *Cochrane Database Systematic Review*, 2004.
6. Project PIaAL. Vital decisions: how Internet users decide what information to trust when they or their loved ones are sick, 2002: wwwintuteacuk/cgi-bin/redirpl?url=http://20721232103/pdfs/PIP_Vital_Decisions_May20 02pdf&handle=20028783.
7. Diaz J, Sciamanna C, Evanelou E, Stamp M, Ferguson T. What types of Internet guidance do patients want from their physicians? *J Gen Intern Med* 2005;**20**:683–5.
8. Ziebland S et al. *BMJ* 2004;**328**:564.

13

Doing your bit

Never doubt that a small group of thoughtful, committed citizens can change the world. Indeed, it's the only thing that ever has.

Margaret Mead[1]

Many consumers now expect, quite rightly, to be involved in making decisions about their healthcare. Sharing the power also means sharing the responsibility. As consumers, we also have an important role to play in improving the quality of healthcare – we cannot leave it all to the health professionals. You can do your bit to improve the quality of healthcare and health information. One important step, as suggested in this book, is to encourage an evidence-based approach to your healthcare. Here are some other suggestions.

Lobbying for more responsible information

If you are confused or dissatisfied with the quality of information, whether on a prescription medicine or in a leaflet handed out by your naturopath or pharmacist, it is your right to take the matter further. Contact the source of the information and ask what evidence is available to support the claims being made. By doing this, you may end up with some useful information, as well as sending the message to organisations that the public will hold them accountable.

If you are not statisfied with the response, you may wish to contact professional or industry associations, regulatory authorities or watchdog groups, such as Consumer Direct (www.consumer direct.gov.uk/), 'Which' (www.which.co.uk/), the National Consumers' Council (www.ncc.org.uk/) or EQUIP – How to complain about an NHS health service (http://www.equip.nhs.uk/support.html) in the UK, or the Australian Consumers' Association (www.choice.com.au) or the Consumers' Health Forum (www.chf.org.au) in Australia. Another useful group of health professionals is Healthy Skepticism (www.healthyskepticism.org), an international watchdog on the pharmaceutical industry. It has documented many instances of unethical or misleading advertising and promotion, and has been successful in having many such breaches rectified. Most countries also have government authorities that monitor or regulate such promotion: in the UK, the Trading Standards Authority (find out more at www.direct.gov.uk/en/RightsAnd Responsibilities/DG_10015892) and in Australia, the Therapeutic Goods Administration (www.tga.gov.au) regulates drugs and devices.

Being part of a trial

> The aim of science is not to open the door to everlasting wisdom,
> but to set a limit on everlasting error.
>
> Albert Brecht, *Galileo*

If there are several treatments and it is unclear which is best, you may wish to consider being part of a trial. Your practitioner may suggest this to you; otherwise you may wish to ask your practitioner whether there are randomised controlled trials that you can enter.

Before a trial is started, the new treatments are tested in a laboratory to ensure, as far as is possible, their safety and effectiveness. They might also have been trialled previously on other people for preliminary information on safety. Throughout the trial details will be collected about your progress and you will be monitored for any adverse effects and, if it is found that a treatment is not in your best interest, you will be removed from the trial and your options discussed. You will receive your care in the same places that standard treatments are given – hospitals, clinics or doctors' offices.

If you decide to participate in a trial, check whether it has been approved by an ethics committee. Ethics committees are run by hospitals and universities and include a range of scientists and community representatives. Among other things, an ethics committee makes sure that, if you enter a trial, you will not have to stop any treatment that is shown to be doing you good. Ethics approval also means that the committee thinks that the benefit-to-harm ratio of the new treatment is no better than existing alternatives. In fact, there is evidence that 50 per cent of trials show the new treatment to be better and 50 per cent show that the old treatment is better. This suggests that, on average, you will have as a good a chance of the best outcome, no matter which arm of the trial you are in. Safety guards are built into trials to ensure that they are stopped as soon as one of the treatments is shown to be better than the other.

What else is in it for you? Joining a trial may offer you the only way of gaining access to a new drug that is not yet generally available. As well, research has shown that practitioners who enter patients in trials generally offer a better standard of care. And, of course, you will be helping to further the march of knowledge as well as improving the prospects for people in the future.

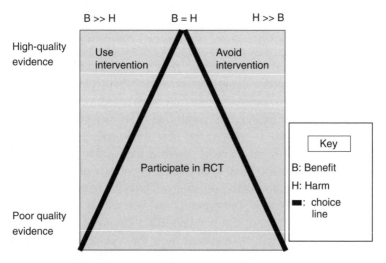

Figure 13.1 When to participate in a randomised trial

It is important to make sure that you understand what the trial entails so that you can give true informed consent to being involved. If it is a trial being run by a pharmaceutical company or other commercial interest, you should ask for an assurance that the results of the trial will be made publicly available and not kept private by the company. Trial results should be made public irrespective of the results; if you are part of a trial that shows a new treatment does not work, you want that to be made known just as much as if the new treatment does work. You may also want to request that a copy of the study results be sent to you as soon as they are available.

The decision to enter a trial depends on the magnitude of the benefits and harms and the quality of evidence as shown in Figure 13.1. Even if the evidence of benefit is not of high quality, you may still choose to use the intervention because it is thought to be free of harms. However, when it is unclear whether the benefits exceed the harms because the evidence is poor, it seems reasonable to be entered into a trial.

Legal issues

It seems right that people should be compensated for serious outcomes stemming from negligence. Therefore, it is important that medicine is challenged and that health practitioners are held accountable. However, we need to remember that serious outcomes may occur even when the appropriate care is given – not all diseases can be cured and nature is uncertain.

There is a growing concern that unrealistic expectations for detecting, diagnosing and treating disease often drive people to sue the practitioner or laboratory for a tragic outcome that may have arisen as an untoward effect of a reasonable process of care. Medicine is not perfect; outcomes are uncertain.

The following is an extract from Professor Fiona Stanley, an eminent Australian epidemiologist:[2]

> Recent litigation has involved women who have claimed that their [cervical] cancers were not picked up by the screening process. These situations are tragic but it is not a failure of the screening

program and it is not negligence on the part of the laboratory – it is expected as part of normal screening activity. These women were the unfortunate few, the very rare cases, the false negatives which occur in any screening program.

The effects of this litigation have been negative in the following ways. Firstly, a marked increase in referrals for slightly abnormal smears. Secondly, major increases to the costs of the program – more repeat tests, more doctors' examinations, more colposcopies, more biopsies and so on. Thirdly, fewer women coming for screening, having been put off the program because of the adverse publicity which is usually damaging to the service and the professions whether they are found eventually liable or not. Fourthly, trained people leaving gynaecology or pathology as they do not like being sued. And lastly, encouragement to search for new technologies or tests which may bring very small gains in terms of increased accuracy but with increases in costs.

It's not beyond the realms of possibility that the increased costs of cervical cancer screening programs could result in them being abandoned. If this community wishes to allow women and their lawyers to sue and be awarded huge damages, then we'll have to accept that there will be more women dying of the disease.

Many doctors feel that they are being encouraged to practise defensive medicine – which means that consumers are more likely to undergo unnecessary tests and treatments – because of growing concern about the threat of legal action.

Such concerns could be allayed if more practitioners and patients used some of the processes in this book to make the best possible decisions jointly. This should improve the quality of care and reduce the number of legal suits against practitioners by making clear what expectations are realistic and encouraging optimal practice, as well as discouraging defensive medicine.

Summary

Everyone has an important part to play in improving the quality of healthcare and health information. One way is to make evidence-based decisions about your healthcare. In addition we can all do the following:

* Lobby for more responsible information by contacting the source of any health information and asking about the available evidence supporting the health claims.

* Offer to be part of a trial when there is uncertainty about which intervention is best. The advantages are:
  - it may be the only way of gaining access to a new drug that is not yet generally available
  - practitioners who enter patients in trials generally offer a better standard of care
  - you will be helping to further the march of knowledge.

* Be better informed about legal issues. Although it seems fair that people should be compensated for serious health effects resulting from negligence, many practitioners are recommending unnecessary tests and treatments because of growing concern about the threat of legal action.

References

1. Mead M. My Quotes Page: www.columbia.edu/~sjp21/quotes.html.
2. The Health Report, Monday, 29 January 1996, Australian Broadcasting Corporation.

14

How to apply the evidence to you and your situation

And finally, here is our summary of how to improve the quality of your healthcare, and sift the good health advice from the masses of bad information that is out there.

Think critically

- **Think probabilistically**: to assess the harms and benefits of health decisions intelligently, you need to know how probable they are, as well as the source and the strength of the probabilistic evidence.
- **Beware anecdotes**: they might sound convincing but are an unreliable source of evidence. For most tests and treatments, you cannot infer a general rule from a single experience – especially if it is not your own.
- **Ask for evidence about outcomes that matter to people**: it's not enough to know that this treatment is effective in rats or at boosting levels of chemical XYZ. Will it improve your quality or quantity of life?
- **It is your right to be informed**: don't be intimidated by the busy schedule or manner of a practitioner. If it is not offered, ask for information that will enable you and your practitioner to choose the best available option. If advertisements, information

leaflets or media reports are unclear or do not provide enough information about the evidence on which they are based, follow them up and request the data.

- **Be sceptical**: advice from those with a vested interest may be biased. Researchers have been known to push a particular aspect of their results. Always assess the quality of the evidence and, if necessary, look elsewhere for more.
- **Newer is not necessarily better**: if a new health product or procedure has not been shown convincingly to be more effective or safer than one that has been around for a while, why use it?
- **Many health problems get better on their own:** this is known as spontaneous remission. After an illness, we may be tempted to believe that a return to good health is the result of a treatment. Of course this may be so, but in many cases it is uncertain whether recovery is the result of an intervention or the body's natural healing process. Because of this, we should be careful not to assume that the therapy caused the cure.
- **Believing is sometimes seeing (the placebo effect)**: when people tell you that such and such a therapy made them feel better or worse, it may not be a result of the chemical or physical effect of the treatment. If we believe that something is helping us, this can affect our recovery. It's common to experience an expected effect after treatment even if the treatment is a placebo or inactive.

Ask key questions

Perhaps our single most important message is the importance of asking the right questions when making decisions about your health. If you have a health problem, the five key questions to ask are:

1. What will happen if I wait and watch?
2. What are my test or treatment options?
3. What are the benefits and harms of these options?
4. How do the benefits and harms weigh up for me?
5. Do I have enough information to make a choice?

Think about all the benefits and harms

Healthcare is being revolutionised by a new movement called evidence-based medicine or evidence-based healthcare. This is encouraging the use of health practices that are based on sound evidence of their benefit exceeding their harm, rather than the opinions of experts or tradition, as has often been the case in the past and often to the detriment of our health. This book aims to help consumers play a part in this revolution and to benefit from it for themselves by learning how to distinguish the good evidence from the bad.

Health evidence can be theoretical (a theory about how or why a treatment ought to work), anecdotal (a report based on one or more individual experiences) or probabilistic (provided by information from many events, allowing predictions of how often something is likely to occur). In health research, the most compelling information comes from probabilistic evidence from studies based on groups of people. Unfortunately, however, not all such studies are of good quality and capable of providing reliable information. The randomised controlled trial (RCT) is the best study design for investigating health interventions, whether it is the effect of a new drug

---

Sources of evidence on the effects of interventions from strong to weak

1. An evidence-based guideline: not all guidelines are based on valid evidence so it is important to check this
2. Randomised controlled trials
3. Non-randomised studies:
   – cohort studies and non-randomised trials
   – population-based case–control studies
   – hospital-based case–control studies
   – other study types
4. Case reports, opinions, clinical impression and opinions of experts

---

or how a new surgical technique compares with an old. Systematic reviews of RCTs combine the results of RCTs to provide the best form of evidence available. Clinical practice guidelines, if evidence based, can provide useful information for consumers and health professionals, but it is important to check the strength of evidence to support particular recommendations.

So if you want more evidence about an option that a practitioner has advised, you should ask (in order of priority):

- **Is there a guideline?** If there is, ask if it is evidence-based. If it is, you and your practitioner should then discuss how to apply the evidence to you. If there is no evidence-based guideline for your problem, the next question is:
- **Is there a systematic review of randomised controlled trials?** If the answer is yes, again you and your practitioner should talk about how best to apply the evidence to your particular problem. If there is no systematic review, you want to know:
- **Are there randomised controlled trials?** If there are, you and your practitioner should discuss how best to use the findings to suit you. If there are no randomised trials, ask:
- **Are there any other studies?** If there are other studies, which fulfil the criteria for good cohort or case–control studies described in Chapter 9, discuss with your practitioner how they apply to you, remembering that the results of these studies are less certain than for RCTs.
- **What are the experts' opinions or are there any case reports?** This last question is on pretty shaky ground due to the lack of evidence being considered. It is really the last resort if the answer to all of the previous questions is definitely NO. If your only option is to rely on this, the general advice would be to use the recommendation if it seems safe, but avoid it if it is likely to have some harm. This applies to interventions where the benefits are unknown and the harm – of varying severity – is known. Many complementary therapies fall into this category where the true benefits are largely unknown and the harms are likely to be small.

Consider how the benefits and harms weigh up for you

Every health decision you make – whether about a therapy, diagnostic or screening test, or change in lifestyle – will involve benefits and harms. However, their importance will be valued differently by different people. Your perceptions of what is important in life will affect how you apply the evidence to your own situation.

Apart from personal preferences, you should also consider your level of risk when applying the evidence to yourself. Factors such as age, gender and family history of disease may be important. And remember 'the five questions' when making important health decisions. Here they are again:

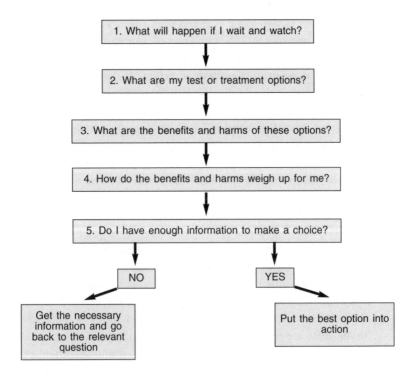

VI

Testing your skill

15

Making sense of health advice

Now it's your turn. See if you can apply what you have learnt about evaluating and applying the validity of information presented in the following examples from the media and research literature.

Do not be put off by jargon that you do not understand, particularly if you are reading the methods and results of studies published in medical journals. The abstracts of many studies are structured to make it easier to assess the quality of the study. In general you can skip the confidence intervals (CIs) if you don't understand them, but, if you want more information on how to interpret confidence intervals, see Chapter 18. Relative risks and odds ratios are also explained more fully in that chapter. Do not be concerned if you do not understand statistical techniques and jargon. Skip over them. Most of the important study flaws have to do with study design rather than statistical errors, so rest assured that, with the help of the validity guides described in Chapters 9 and 10, you should be able to make good sense of the majority of health information, without having to understand the details of statistical methods.

Our appraisal of the evidence is included, but try not to look at this until you've made your judgement.

Please note that the examples in this chapter have been selected so that we can look at their method and validity; they do not necessarily represent the most up-to-date information on a particular topic, and should not be used to inform your own decisions.

Remember, when assessing evidence on TREATMENTS, that you want to know:

1. Is there an evidence-based guideline or systematic review of randomised trials?
2. Is the evidence relevant to your needs?
   - Are the outcomes person centred rather than theoretical? (What should work in theory doesn't always work in practice.)
   - Does the evidence describe both benefits and harms and say how likely they are to occur?
   - Does the evidence describe how treatments compare with other appropriate options?
3. Is the evidence reliable?
   - Is there a systematic review of randomised controlled trials or evidence-based guideline?
   - Are there randomised controlled trials?
   - Are there any non-randomised studies (in order of priority):
     - cohort and non-randomised trials?
     - population-based case–control studies?
     - hospital-based case–control studies?
     - other types of studies?
   - Are there any case reports or opinions?

When assessing evidence on CAUSES of disease or conditions you want to know:

1. Is the evidence about a causal relationship from a reliable source?
   - Is there a systematic review of randomised controlled trials?
   - Are there randomised controlled trials?
   - Are there any non-randomised studies (in order of priority):
     - cohort and non-randomised trials?
     - population-based case–control studies?
     - hospital-based case–control studies?
     - other types of studies?
   - Are there any case reports or opinions?
2. Did exposure to the supposed cause occur before the outcome?

3. Is there a strong relationship between the supposed cause and the outcome?
4. Does the risk of the outcome increase as the dose or length of time of the supposed cause increases?
5. Is there any other explanation for the relationship between the supposed cause and the outcome?
6. Are there other studies showing the same results?
7. Does the 'cause-and-effect' relationship make sense?

Example 1: Making sense of a study

A study on the effects of breastfeeding on pain experienced by babies. 'Analgesic effect of breastfeeding in term neonates: a randomised controlled trial.' By Ricardo Carbajal, Soocramanien Veerapen, Sophie Couderc, Myriam Jugie, Yves Ville. Published in the *British Medical Journal*, volume 326, 4 January, 2003.[1]

Abstract

OBJECTIVES: To investigate whether breastfeeding is effective for pain relief during venepuncture in term neonates and compare any effect with that of oral glucose combined with a pacifier.

DESIGN: Randomised controlled trial.

Participants: 180 term newborn infants undergoing venepuncture; 45 in each group.

Interventions: during venepuncture infants were either breastfed (group 1), held in their mother's arms without breastfeeding (group 2), given 1 ml of sterile water as placebo (group 3) or given 1 ml of 30 per cent glucose followed by pacifier (group 4). Video recordings of the procedure were assessed by two observers blinded to the purpose of the study.

Main outcome measures: pain-related behaviours evaluated with two acute pain rating scales: the Douleur Aiguë Nouveau-né scale (range 0–10) and the premature infant pain profile scale (range 0–18).

RESULTS: Median pain scores (interquartile range) for breastfeeding, held in mother's arms, placebo and 30 per cent glucose plus pacifier groups were 1 (0–3), 10 (8.5–10), 10 (7.5–10) and 3

(0–5) with the Douleur Aiguë Nouveau–né scale, and 4.5 (2.25–8), 13 (10.5–15), 12 (9–13) and 4 (1–6) with the premature infant pain profile scale. Analysis of variance showed significantly different median pain scores (p <0.0001) among the groups. There were significant reductions in both scores for the breastfeeding and glucose plus pacifier groups compared with the other two groups (p <0.0001, two-tailed Mann–Whitney U tests between groups). The difference in Douleur Aiguë Nouveau-né scores between breastfeeding and glucose plus pacifier groups was not significant (p = 0.16).

CONCLUSIONS: Breastfeeding effectively reduces response to pain during minor invasive procedure in term neonates.

Our appraisal

This shows just how straightforward it can be to appraise a structured abstract. You don't have to be a scientist!

- It is controlled, and compares four groups – breastfeeding, being held in mother's arms without feeding, sterile water (control), sugar followed by a pacifier.
- It is randomised.
- It is a double-blind trial. This tells you that the babies, not surprisingly, were unaware of which group they were in, and the investigators listening to the tapes were unaware of which babies were given which intervention.
- There was complete follow-up.

This is a randomised controlled trial, the best type of study for evaluating the effects of an intervention. It meets the validity criteria, and shows that breastfeeding reduces crying in babies when they have a painful procedure such as having blood taken. In addition, it shows that sugar followed by a pacifier was also an effective strategy to reduce crying but not as effective as breastfeeding. We should be careful, however, when applying these results more generally. As with most studies, not all the important issues will have been assessed. For example, this study does not report on the mothers' stress levels if holding or breastfeeding their baby while a blood test is being taken.

Example 2: Should a woman in her 40s have screening mammography?

As a 40-year-old woman, you are concerned with maintaining your health. You see a sticker advertising **Breast Screening for Women 50 and over . . . it's FREE!**

While taking your son to the GP, you pick up a brochure entitled **Early Detection, the Best Protection**, which tells you about the National Program for the Detection of Breast Cancer. It tells you that 1 in 14 women will develop breast cancer in her lifetime and that over 70 per cent of breast cancers occur in women over 50. Further on you read that the target population for mammographic screening is 50–69 years, and that screening in this age group reduces deaths from breast cancer. It goes on to say that the evidence of benefit is not strong enough to recommend routine screening for women in the 40- to 49-year age group and adds: **(Women in this age group can be screened if they wish.)**

Based on this information, how do you make the decision about whether you should be screened? You phone your local mammography clinic who send you a leaflet. You find a table showing the probability of developing breast cancer (incidence), and dying from breast cancer, at different age intervals. Here you see that your risk of developing breast cancer during the decade 40–49 years is about 14 cancers per 1000 women, and your risk of death from breast cancer is about 2.5 deaths per 1000 women. The risks increase with age.

You feel that there is still more you need to know. In particular, you want to know whether the risk of death is reduced by regular screening in your age group and what the possible harms are. You have read the chapter on finding the best evidence and using 'Google' you find an online decision aid about breast cancer screening in women aged 40–49 years (www.mammogram.med.usyd. edu.au).[2] This shows you that the risk of dying from breast cancer between ages 40 and 49 changes from 2.5 per 1000 women *without* screening to 2.0 per 1000 women *with* screening. The decision aid also tells you about the accuracy of screening and the chance of each possible outcome. It explains that over the same decade of 2-yearly screening:

- 21 women are diagnosed with breast cancer over the next 10 years
- 12 women have their cancer detected by screening
- 9 women develop symptoms and are diagnosed with breast cancer between screening mammograms
- 239 women have extra tests after an abnormal mammogram. The extra tests will show that these women don't have breast cancer. Aside from the inconvenience of attending for these tests, some women will worry long after they have had them
- 740 women are correctly reassured that they do not have breast cancer.

Our appraisal

Weighing up the benefits and the harms of screening should be done on an individual basis. Most people believe that screening for cancer is something worthwhile but it's important to understand that these tests are not perfect. Some, but not all, cancers will be detected by screening. Sometimes test results can be falsely positive and invasive follow-up tests might be performed on a completely healthy person. Different people will place different values on the benefits and risks of screening. For some the chance that one life might be saved over 10 years is highly regarded. For others, it might not seem a substantial benefit for them. Many women won't mind having extra follow-up tests for an abnormal mammogram provided that they get the 'all clear' in the end. Others will be annoyed that this extra stress, expense and inconvenience have been caused. There's no right or wrong answer. Everyone will be different.

Evidence-based decision aids to help you weigh up the benefits and risks of screening are available through the Sydney Health Decision Group (mammography in 40- to 49-year-old women at www.mammogram.med.usyd.edu.au and FOBT [faecal occult blood test] screening for bowel cancer at www.cancerscreeningdecision.org).

Example 3: Product information – Blackmores Hyperiforte 1800 (St John's wort)

You are feeling anxious and depressed and have spoken to your practitioner about how you are feeling. He says you could take antidepressants, but your symptoms are relatively mild and may not warrant the risk of side effects. He suggests that you try St John's wort (Hypericon) which is available from chemists or health food shops without a prescription and seems safe. When you are next at the shops, you find a bottle of St John's wort, and are surprised to find a reference to an article in a medical journal on the product information on the side of the bottle. It reads:

> Blackmores Hyperiforte 1800 helps relieve nervous tension, stress and mild anxiety. Hyperiforte 1800 is formulated to replicate the dose used in clinical trials, where it was demonstrated to be as effective as prescription drugs but with fewer side effects.
>
> *Vorbach et al.*[3]

You could find the abstract of the article on PubMed (www.ncbi.nlm.nih.gov/PubMed), which is free to use, but it might be more sensible to see whether there is any more recent and complete information. You look at the Cochrane Library home page (www.thecochranelibrary.com) and a search for 'wort' finds the following:

St John's Wort for Depression Linde K, Mulrow CD Date of most recent substantive amendment: 25/02/2005

Plain language summary

Available evidence suggests that several specific extracts of St John's wort may be effective for treating mild to moderate depression, although the data are not fully convincing.

Extracts of St John's wort (botanical name *Hypericum perforatum L.*) are prescribed widely for the treatment of depression. They seem more effective than placebo and similarly effective as standard antidepressants for treating mild to moderate depressive symptoms.

Beneficial effects for treating major depression appear minimal. Side effects are usually minor and uncommon. However, as extracts of St John's wort can influence adverse effects of other drugs, patients should consult their physicians before using St John's wort. The results of this review apply only to the preparations tested in trials; the content of marketed preparations might vary considerably from those tested in trials.

Linde et al.[4]

Our appraisal

This is a good systematic review. There are many trials, showing St John's wort to be beneficial when compared with placebo, and that it may be as effective as standard antidepressants, but with fewer side effects. You may decide that it is worth taking.

Example 4: Keyhole or open surgery for a hernia? Which is best for me?

You are a middle-aged man with a swelling in your groin that your doctor tells you is an inguinal hernia. Although there is no urgency, you decide to have it operated on because it is uncomfortable and interferes with your work and leisure activities. While chatting to a friend, he tells you he also had a similar operation a while ago and noticed that there was some press coverage about inguinal hernias at that time. After some searching among some old papers in his filing cabinet, he finds an article from a newspaper which reads:

It was business as usual for Dr Michael Aroney as he performed keyhole surgery to repair a hernia on a 62-year-old man injured at work.

The operation, which Dr Aroney performed yesterday at the Holroyd Private Hospital, Guildford, is a typical example of the problems facing the health funds.

The treatment – the finest available – means the man will be able to return to work within two weeks. But this comes at a price. The operation will cost nearly $1,000 more than conventional surgery, which would have kept the patient out of work for at least six weeks.

'Medicine is not cheap,' said Dr Aroney. 'It comes at a price.

'People have high expectations, and those high expectations require high-tech medicine, and that does not come cheaply.'

Health funds are keen to introduce a system where decisions to operate in the most modern manner possible will come under more rigorous scrutiny. For example, should Dr Aroney have used cheaper, more conventional surgical techniques?

Was surgery even necessary? It would have been possible for the man to have been prescribed a truss at virtually no cost. Such a system was not mentioned in yesterday's report, but it may not be far off.

The Government has not ruled out further inquiries into how to control costs in hospitals, even to the extent of deciding which is the most appropriate and most effective treatment.

The minister has guaranteed that the final decision will be with doctors, but not necessarily the surgeon performing the surgery.

Dr Aroney, like many doctors, believes it would be the wrong way to go, saying:

'Doctors jealously guard the fact that they have a patient–doctor relationship and they are directly responsible to their patients, rather than to a third party.'

Marion Downey – *Sydney Morning Herald*, Page 6, Friday,
11 April 1997. Section: News and Features

You want to have some say in the operation you have, particularly as it is important to you to return to work soon as you work on your own and have difficulty in taking time off. You chat to your doctor about surgeons and ask which surgeons are best and whether any of the ones whom she recommends has experience with 'laparo-scopic' (keyhole) surgery for hernia. (As discussed in Chapter 4, technical expertise hangs on three broad criteria: qualification to perform the procedure, experience in performing the procedure, and being part of a quality assurance scheme or some similar credentialing programme.) You also ask what the evidence is that keyhole surgery does as well as open surgery. Your doctor checks for systematic reviews on the Cochrane Library online while you are there and finds one: McCormack K, Scott N, G. P, Ross, S and Grant A, Laporoscopic techniques versus open techniques for inguinal hernia repair. There was no plain language summary at the time this book was published.[5]

Abstract

OBJECTIVES: To compare minimal access laparoscopic mesh techniques with open techniques.

SEARCH STRATEGY: We searched Medline, Embase and the Cochrane Central Controlled Trials Registry for relevant randomised controlled trials. The reference list of identified trials, journal supplements, relevant book chapters and conference proceedings were searched for further relevant trials. Through the EU Hernia Trialists Collaboration (EUHTC) communication took place with authors of identified randomised controlled trials to ask for information on any other recent and ongoing trials known to them.

SELECTION CRITERIA: All published and unpublished randomised controlled trials and quasi-randomised controlled trials comparing laparoscopic groin hernia repair with open groin hernia repair were eligible for inclusion.

DATA COLLECTION AND ANALYSIS: Individual patient data (IPID) were obtained, where possible, from the responsible trialist for all eligible studies. Where IPD was unavailable additional aggregate data were sought from trialists and published aggregate data checked and verified by the trialists. Where possible, time to event analysis for hernia recurrence and return to usual activities were performed on an intention to treat principle. The main analyses were based on all trials. Sensitivity analyses based on the data source and trial quality were also performed. Predefined subgroup analyses based on recurrent hernias, bilateral hernias and femoral hernias were also carried out.

MAIN RESULT: Forty-one eligible trials of laparoscopic versus open groin hernia repair were identified involving 7161 participants (with individual patient data available for 4165). Meta-analysis was performed, using IDP where possible. Operation times for laparoscopic repair were longer and there was a higher risk of rare serious complications. Return to usual activities was faster, and there was less persisting pain and numbness. Hernia recurrence was less common than after open non-mesh repair but not different to open mesh methods.

AUTHORS' CONCLUSIONS: The review showed that laparoscopic repair takes longer and has a more serious complication rate in respect of visceral (especially bladder) and vascular injuries, but recovery is quicker with less persisting pain and numbness. Reduced hernia recurrence rates of around 30–50 per cent were related to the use of mesh rather than the method of mesh placement.

Our appraisal

This systematic review combines the results of 41 randomised trials that involved over 7000 people in total. It tells you that laparoscopic repair allows you to get back to work quicker and that persistent pain and numbness are less likely. However, the operation takes longer to perform and rare serious complications of the bladder and blood vessels are more likely. Hernia recurrence rates are about the same as open-mesh surgery. We had to look into the main part of the review to find the complication rates for laparoscopic repair. Although the abstract doesn't mention it, the laparoscopic complication rate is about 87 per 1000 operations with blood clots, 15 per 1000 with wound infections and 3 in 1000 with bladder damage. Compare this to open-mesh complications rates and you have 107 blood clots per 1000, 31 wound infections per 1000 and fewer than 1 per 1000 cases of bladder damage.

Your doctor explains that you need to weigh up the slightly higher chance of more serious complications against the better short-term outcomes including earlier return to work. As early return to work is critical to you at the moment, you decide to have a laparoscopic repair if there is a surgeon in your town who has experience with the operation.

CHAPTER 15

Example 5: Do mobile phones cause brain cancer?

Mobile phone cancer link rejected. BBC News, 30 August 2005:
http://news.bbc.co.uk/1/hi/health/4196762.stm

> Mobile phone use does not raise the risk of cancer, at least in the
> first 10 years of use, the largest investigation to date shows.
>
> Some past studies had suggested an increased risk of acoustic
> neuroma – a tumour of the nerve connecting the ear and the brain
> – but others did not.
>
> The latest Institute of Cancer Research work includes data from five
> European countries and more than 4000 people.
>
> Expert advice is still to limit mobile phone use as a precautionary
> measure.
>
> There are more than one billion mobile phone users worldwide.
>
> Longer follow-up is needed to check that health problems do not
> arise with many more years of use, the researchers say in the *British
> Journal of Cancer.*
>
> An independent group for the UK government, led by Sir William
> Stewart, that looked into the safety of mobile phones in the late
> 1990s also concluded that mobile phones did not appear to harm
> health.
>
> However, the group said that there was evidence that radiation from
> mobile phones could potentially cause adverse health effects, and
> therefore a 'precautionary approach' to their use should be adopted.

Precautions

> The government currently advises mobile phone users to keep their
> call times short.
>
> And children under the age of 16 should use mobile phones for
> essential calls only, because their head and nervous systems may
> still be developing.

The latest data from the UK, Denmark, Finland, Norway and Sweden included 678 people with acoustic neuroma and 3553 without this form of tumour.

This revealed no relationship between the risk of acoustic neuroma and the number of years for which the mobile phones had been used, the time since first use, total hours of use or total number of calls.

Nor was there any link with analogue or digital phones or whether or not a hands-free kit was used.

On balance, the evidence suggests that there is no substantial risk of acoustic neuroma in the first decade of use – but the possibility of some effect after longer periods remains open, the researchers concluded.

Senior investigator Professor Anthony Swerdlow said: 'Whether there are longer-term risks remains unknown, reflecting the fact that this is a relatively recent technology.'

Dr Michael Clark from the Health Protection Agency said: 'This is good news but we still need to be a bit cautious.'

Dr Julie Sharp, senior science information officer at Cancer Research UK, said: 'This study provides further evidence that using mobile phones does not increase the risk of brain tumours.

'However, it is important that researchers continue to monitor phone users over the coming years as mobiles are still a relatively new invention.'

The research is part of a bigger study that will be published next year.

A Swedish study identified an increased risk of acoustic neuromas among people who had used mobile phones for 10 years or more.

People have been concerned that the radiofrequency from phones might cause cancers, despite the absence of a known biological mechanism for this.

Our appraisal

The evidence about the relationship should be from a reliable source and the best study type

This news article doesn't tell us what type of study the claim is based on, only that it has been conducted across five European countries. If you go to PubMed and type in (acoustic neuroma) AND (mobile phone) AND 2005, you will find that this is describing a population-based case–control study in which the prior use of mobile phones is measured in people with acoustic neuroma and in a sample of the general population.[6] Randomised trials are impractical because one could not randomise people to use mobile phones. Cohort studies, the next best design, would be very difficult to do because acoustic neuromas are quite rare, only occurring in about 6 out of every 100,000 people each year. This means that a cohort study would require follow-up of millions of mobile phone users and non-users over a decade or more. Population-based case–control studies are therefore likely to be about as good as it gets. You can read more about cohort and case–control studies in Chapter 10.

The exposure to the supposed cause should occur before the outcome

From reading this news story, it seems that they asked all participants about mobile phone use over the preceding 10 years. Although this does record mobile phone exposure *before* developing an acoustic neuroma, it is prone to bias because people's recollections about use over such a long period of time might not be very accurate. It might be that people who have a brain tumour tend to over-recall higher phone usage in hindsight compared with those who don't have a brain tumour.

There should be a strong relationship between the supposed cause and the outcome

The study didn't find any overall association between mobile phone use and acoustic neuroma at least within 10 years.

There should be a dose–response or exposure–response relationship between the supposed cause and outcome, that is, the greater the exposure, the more likely someone is to get a disease
The study looked at the number of hours of mobile phone use and the number of years of mobile phone use and did not find any relationship to cancer risk.

There should not be any other factors that could explain the relationship
Actually as we don't know much about the cause of brain tumours, it is difficult to know whether other factors could play a part in the development of acoustic neuroma.

The same results should be shown in several studies
Looking at PubMed by typing in (mobile phone) AND (brain cancer) we can see that the interphone study involving the five countries that this BBC item refers to is the main study that has been conducted. It has shown that there is also no link between mobile phone use for less than 10 years and gliomas (another type of brain tumour).[7]

The relationship should make sense
This has been addressed at the end of the news item where it states that people's concerns have not been based on a known biological cause.

The bottom line on this question is that there is reasonable evidence that mobile phone use does *not* increase your risk of brain cancer within 10 years. The type of study design is a population-based case–control study, which is the best study type that is feasible for a rare condition. As the BBC has suggested, mobile phone technology is new and we don't know about potential risks after 10 years of use.

Applying the principles we have set out in this book, you will hopefully be weighing up the benefits and convenience of mobile phone use in your own situation against the evidence to date. Researchers have not shown any link so far and it's important to bear in mind that brain cancers are less common than many others.

References

1. Carbajal R, Veerapen S, Couderc S, Jugie M, Ville Y. Analgesic effect of breast feeding in term neonates: randomised controlled trial. *BMJ* 2003;**326**:13.
2. Barratt A, Howard K, Irwig L, Salkeld G, Houssami N. Model of outcomes of screening mammography: information to support informed choices. *BMJ* 2005: doi:10.1136/bmj.38398.469479.8F.
3. Vorbach E, Hubner W, Arnoldt K. Effectiveness and tolerance of the hypericum extract LI 160 in comparison with imipramine: randomized double-blind study with 135 outpatients. *J Geriatr Psychiatry Neurol* 1994;**7**(suppl 1):S19–23.
4. Linde K, Mulrow C, Berner M, Egger M. St John's wort for depression. *Cochrane Database of Systematic Reviews*, 2005; Apr 18(2):CD000448.
5. McCormack K, Scott N, Go P, Ross S, Grant A. Laparoscopic techniques versus open techniques for inguinal hernia repair. *Cochrane Database of Systematic Reviews*, 2003;1:CD001785.
6. Schoemaker M, Swerdlow A, Ahlbom A et al. Mobile phone use and risk of acoustic neuroma: results of the Interphone case-control study in five North European countries. *Br J Cancer* 2005;**93**:842–8.
7. Lahkola A, Auvinen A, Raitanen J et al. Mobile phone use and risk of glioma in 5 North European countries. *Int J Cancer* 2007;**120**:1769–75.

16

Is this a useful diagnostic test?

The next three chapters have been provided for those readers who really want to understand and learn some basic epidemiological skills. You may be a health consumer who has really found this book interesting and wants to go a bit further. You may be a health practitioner or practitioner in training and want to brush up on some skills in evidence-based practice. Whoever you are, if you are the sort of person who does not like numbers, you might want to skip over this part.

Sensitivity and specificity of a diagnostic test

*   *Sensitivity* indicates the probability that the test will accurately pick up disease when there truly is disease.
*   *Specificity* indicates the probability that the test will accurately detect 'NO disease' when the disease is truly absent.

To illustrate these, imagine I have a bag of toffees, some of which are liquorice flavoured (L) and some of which are not (NOT-L). L and NOT-L toffees have a slightly different shape so it's easy for me (or so I believe) to feel which is which without looking. To see how accurate I am at detecting which are which, I try it out.

This is the result: of 100 L toffees, my hand correctly calls 80 of them L toffees. Of 100 NOT-L toffees, my hand correctly calls 90 of them NOT-L toffees.

In technical jargon, if I consider my hand as a diagnostic test, it has a sensitivity of 80 per cent (the proportion of L toffees that I correctly identified) and a specificity of 90 per cent (the proportion of NOT-L toffees that I correctly identified).

Pre-test and post-test probability

Now if I put my hand in a bag of toffees and say 'This is a liquorice toffee', what are my chances of being correct? Well, I cannot tell what my chances are of being right unless I know something about the existing probability of finding a liquorice toffee. This is referred to as the *pre-test probability* of an L toffee. For example, if there are no L toffees in that bag, all of those that I call L would be wrong calls. On the other hand, if the bag contains only L toffees, all those that I call L will be correct calls (and, of course, any 'NOT-L' calls would be wrong!). So even though I may know the sensitivity and specificity of my hand as a test, I need more information to interpret the test result.

Clearly the interpretation of the test depends on what percentage of the toffees in the bag were L or NOT-L before I put my hand in it. Put another way, it depends on the pre-test probability of a

Table 16.1 My probability of correctly detecting L toffees: pre-test probability of 25 per cent

	Truly L toffees	Truly NOT-L toffees	Total	Probability of a toffee being L
I think that they are L toffees	80	30	110	Post-test prob. for a positive test = 80/110 = 73%
I think that they are NOT-L toffees	20	270	290	Post-test probability for a negative test = 20/290 = 7%
Total	100	300	400	Pre-test probability = 100/400 = 25%

toffee being L. Now if I knew that, working out the result of my test would be easy. Here are a few numerical examples of the toffee test:

Suppose I have a bag of 400 toffees, of which 25 per cent (i.e. 100 toffees) are L. If I have been told that this is the case, I can apply the sensitivity and specificity of my hand to this set of information as shown in Table 16.1.

In Table 16.1, the sensitivity is 80 per cent (80/100) and the specificity 90 per cent (270/300). I know this from applying my known sensitivity and specificity in detecting L and NOT-L toffees as described earlier. Now, if I put my hand in and detect a toffee as L the probability of being correct is 73 per cent (80/110). If I think that it is NOT-L, of course, there is still a chance that it actually is L – a 7 per cent (20/290) chance to be precise.

Now, let's imagine that I am given another bag of 400 toffees and, this time, 75 per cent of them are L toffees instead of 25 per cent. Needless to say, the sensitivity and specificity of my hand (remember my hand is the diagnostic test) remain the same, so this time the table would be as shown in Table 16.2.

Now, if I say I think that a toffee is L, I will be correct 96 per cent of the time and, if I identify it as NOT-L, there is a 40 per cent

Table 16.2 My probability of correctly detecting L toffees: pre-test probability of 75 per cent

	Truly L toffees	Truly NOT-L toffees	Total	Probability of a toffee being L
I think that they are L toffees	240	10	250	Post-test probability for a positive test = 240/250 = 96%
I think that they are NOT-L toffees	60	90	150	Post-test probability for a negative test = 60/150 = 40%
Total	300	100	400	Pre-test probability = 300/400 = 75%

chance that it turns out to be L, which translates to a 60 per cent chance that I will be right in my call.

In medical jargon, then, the PRE-TEST PROBABILITY is the probability that L toffees are in the bag before I put my hand in it or, more appropriately, the probability that there really is disease before a diagnostic test is carried out. The POST-TEST PROBABILITY if the test turns out to be POSITIVE is the probability that I will detect an L toffee when it truly is one, whereas the POST-TEST PROBABILITY if the test is NEGATIVE is the probability of it really being L when I judge it not to be. In terms of disease, it is the probability of the existence of disease when the test detects no disease.

Table 16.3 Summary of all the above information

Pre-test probability of L (%)	Post-test probability of a positive test (%)	Post-test probability of a negative test (%)
0	0	0
25	73	7
75	96	40
100	100	100

In summary, the post-test probability of disease given a diagnostic test result depends on the sensitivity and specificity of the test AND on the pre-test probability. There is no such thing as being absolutely certain of what a test result means; it varies from one patient to another depending on his or her pre-test probability. For instance, a positive HIV test in an intravenous drug user means something different to a positive HIV test on a blood donation from, say, a nun. For the drug user the pre-test probability may be appreciable and a positive test is likely to indicate HIV. In the nun, on the other hand, the pre-test probability is close to zero and any positive test is likely to be a false positive.

Note that the post-test probabilities for negative and positive tests straddle the pre-test probability – that is, a positive test increases the probability of disease above the pre-test level, whereas a negative test decreases it to below the pre-test level. When you do choose to have a further diagnostic test, use of pre-test and post-test probabilities will tell you how the test results affect your chances of having the disease.

To give you some examples, screening mammography has a sensitivity of about 85 per cent in women over 50 and about 70 per cent in women aged between 40 and 49.[1] Specificity is about 95 per cent – that is, about 5 per cent of women without cancer will require some further investigation. Ultrasound has a sensitivity of about 85 per cent and a specificity of 90 per cent in detecting blockage in the arteries to the brain.[2] However, ultrasound has a sensitivity of only about 60 per cent and a specificity of 97 per cent for detecting clots in the veins in the legs after operations.[3] Of course, one can also assess the accuracy of symptoms and the signs. For example, if you are admitted to hospital with possible appendicitis, the pain in the bottom right part of your abdomen has a sensitivity of 81 per cent and a specificity of 53 per cent.[4]

Like you, many practitioners find this complex. This type of information may not have been part of their medical training. Consequently, you are likely to find the answers about your pre-test and post-test probabilities less satisfactory than answers about the effects of treatments.

References

1. Kerlikowske K, Grady D, Sickles EA, Ernster V. Effect of age, breast density, and family history on the sensitivity of first screening mammography. *JAMA* 1996; **276(1)**:33–38.
2. Blakeley DD, Oddone EZ, Hasselblad V, et al. Noninvasive carotid artery testing: a meta-analytic review. *Annals of Internal Medicine* 1995; **122(5)**:360–367.
3. Wells PS, Lansing AW, Davidson BL, et al. Accuracy of ultrasound for the diagnosis of deep venous thrombosis in asymptomatic patients after orthopaedic surgery: a meta-analysis. *Annals of Internal Medicine* 1995; **122(1)**:47–53.
4. Wagner JM, McKinney WP, Carpenter JC, et al. Does this patient have appendicitis? *JAMA* 1996; **276**:1584–1594.

17

Decision thresholds

Suppose that you have a cough that has persisted for several days. Your doctor tells you that it should be treated with antibiotics if it is a bacterial infection. You could:

- wait to see if it clears up without treatment
- treat with antibiotics in case there is a bacterial chest infection
- have a test to establish whether there is a bacterial chest infection.

How you decide goes something like this: if the probability that the cough is caused by a bacterial chest infection is 0 per cent, you clearly would not have antibiotics. On the other hand, if the probability is 100 per cent, you would take antibiotics. Anywhere between these extremes a diagnostic test would help to determine the chance that the infection is bacterial. So why not just go ahead and have a test? For two reasons: first, there are almost always harms associated with tests and, second, a test does not guarantee absolute certainty about the diagnosis. One way of dealing with this uncertainty is to use *the decision threshold*, which is illustrated by the following example.

Say your practitioner tells you that the probability of your having a bacterial infection is less than 10 per cent. You might decide to wait a few days to see if you feel better without any treatment. Ten per cent may be your threshold below which the harms of a test or treatment outweigh its potential benefit. If, on the other hand, your practitioner thinks there is a very high probability of a bacterial infection, say above 90 per cent, a course of antibiotics may be the best way to go. Ninety per cent, in this case, may be your threshold above which treatment is advisable without undergoing a test. This is because the benefit of treatment outweighs the potential harms of not treating, of the test itself and of the delay while waiting for a test result.

But what if your practitioner tells you that the probability of bacterial infection is about 50 per cent? This is between your thresholds for doing nothing (below 10 per cent) or taking antibiotics (above 90 per cent). In this case, having a diagnostic test to establish the real cause of the cough may be a good choice. These concepts are summarised in the Figure below.

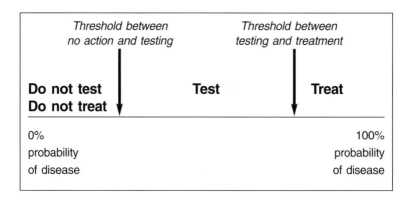

To summarise, using the *decision threshold* method of deciding the best course of action requires that you and your practitioner have an estimate of your chance of having a particular disease, and comparing that to thresholds below which it would be best not to treat and above which it would be best to treat. Only between these thresholds can a test be of any help.

CHAPTER 17

How do you or your practitioner decide exactly where the thresholds are? It really depends on the benefits and harms of treating or not treating. Suppose, for example, a safe and effective treatment exists for a disease that you may have. This would lower the threshold above which to treat because there would be less reason to avoid treatment. By the same token, if the only diagnostic test available is invasive (an aggressive procedure) and not very accurate, you may decide either to 'wait and watch' or to treat (just in case) and avoid the test.

18

Relative risk, relative and absolute risk reduction, number needed to treat and confidence intervals

Relative and absolute risks

How do you interpret the results of a randomised controlled trial? A common measure of a treatment is to look at the frequency of bad outcomes of a disease in the group being treated compared with those who were not treated. For instance, supposing that a well-designed randomised controlled trial in children with a particular disease found that 20 per cent of the control group developed bad outcomes, compared with only 12 per cent of those receiving treatment. Should you agree to give this treatment to your child? Without knowing more about the adverse effects of the therapy, it appears to reduce some of the bad outcomes of the disease. But is its effect meaningful?

This is where you need to consider the risk of treatment versus no treatment. In healthcare, risk refers to the probability of a bad outcome in people with the disease.

Absolute risk reduction (ARR) – also called risk difference (RD) – is the most useful way of presenting research results to help your decision-making. In this example, the ARR is 8 per cent (20 per cent - 12 per cent = 8 per cent). This means that, if 100 children were treated, 8 would be prevented from developing bad outcomes. Another way of expressing this is the number needed to treat (NNT).

If 8 children out of 100 benefit from treatment, the NNT for one child to benefit is about 13 (100 ÷ 8 = 12.5).

For technical reasons, some other measures are often used. The relative risk (RR) of a bad outcome in a group given intervention is a proportional measure estimating the size of the effect of a treatment compared with other interventions or no treatment at all. It is the proportion of bad outcomes in the intervention group divided by the proportion of bad outcomes in the control group. In this hypothetical case, the RR is 0.6 (12 per cent ÷ 20 per cent = 0.6).

When a treatment has an RR greater than 1, the risk of a bad outcome is increased by the treatment; when the RR is less than 1, the risk of a bad outcome is decreased, meaning that the treatment is likely to do good. For example, when the RR is 2.0 the chance of a bad outcome is twice as likely to occur with the treatment as without it, whereas an RR of 0.5 means that the chance of a bad outcome is twice as likely to occur without the intervention. When the RR is exactly 1, the risk is unchanged. For example, a report may state 'The relative risk of blindness in people given drug T was 1.5'. This shows that the drug increased the risk of blindness. Another measure that is used is the odds ratio. For practical purposes, assume that the odds ratio is the same as the relative risk. Sometimes the outcome is a good one and the interpretation of relative risk is the opposite of what we have just outlined.

Relative risk reduction (RRR) tells you by how much the treatment reduced the risk of bad outcomes relative to the control group who did not have the treatment. In the previous example, the relative risk reduction of fever and rash in the group of the children on the intervention was 40 per cent (1 − 0.6 = 0.4 or 40 per cent).

Table 18.1 Percentage with poor outcomes

% Control with poor outcomes	% intervention with poor outcomes	RR	RRR	ARR (%)	NNT
60	40	0.67	0.33	20	5
30	20	0.6	0.33	10	10
15	10	0.67	0.33	5	20
3	1	0.67	0.33	2	50

The RR (and therefore the RRR) is often the same in people irrespective of their level of risk, which means that the ARR will be greatest in those at greatest risk, as shown in Table 18.1. The greater your risk, the more you stand to gain from the intervention.

Confidence intervals

Confidence intervals (CIs) aim to give you an idea of how confident you can be about a study's estimate of a treatment's effects. Even when a study is of impeccable quality, the results may have happened by chance. Statisticians deal with this uncertainly by doing some nifty calculations to determine how confident one can be about the results, which give us the confidence interval. The narrower the range, the more precise the study's estimates, and the more confident you can be that it is a 'real' finding and not due to chance.

This is usually expressed in terms of a 95 per cent confidence interval (95%CI), which represents the range of results within which we can be 95 per cent certain that the true answer lies.

As an illustration of how confidence intervals can help, imagine that you are doing a study investigating whether there is gender bias in the method used by a university to choose its students. If there were no such bias you would expect 50 per cent of its students to be men and 50 per cent to be women. Supposing that you check a small sample, say 10 students, and found 4 of them were men. How sure can you be that this is a true reflection of the student population? Statistical calculations show that you can be 95 per cent certain that the true quota of men in the entire university population is somewhere between 12 and 74 per cent. This is an unhelpfully wide range.

But supposing you randomly sample 100 students and find that 40 are men. Statistical calculations show that you can be 95 per cent certain that the true quota of men in the entire university population is somewhere between 30 and 50 per cent – a narrower range.

Imagine also that you randomly examined a large sample of 1000 students, of whom 400 were men. The 95%CI would be from 37 per cent to 43 per cent – a much narrower range showing a very high level of confidence that this represents a true reflection of the gender ratio in the university.

In the sample of 10 students, finding four men is compatible with our expected value for society at large – 50 per cent males and 50 per cent females. In the group of 1000 students finding that only 40 per cent are men is not expected. The result from this large sample is statistically significant, which means that the disparity between the observed 40 per cent and the expected 50 per cent is real – that is, it is very unlikely to have arisen by chance. In the sample of 100 students, the upper end of the confidence interval is just on the expected value of 50 per cent and therefore just statistically significant.

The same principle applies to studies investigating treatments, except that we might be looking at the relative risks of a poor outcome in the group receiving the intervention compared with the control group.

Useful sources of health advice

'Ensuring access' means making information both comprehensible and available to others. These two elements need to be of equal concern.

Hilda Bastian, The Power of Sharing Knowledge

As new health information sources are constantly being created, we have chosen *not* to list website addresses for you here but have listed some names of organisations and online resources that might be of interest. To find these you can type the names or titles into search engines such as 'Google' or 'Yahoo' or you could visit our 'Smart Health Choices' website for current links to evidence-based online information. http://www.health.usyd.edu.au/shdg/resources/ebooks.php/

Evidence-based healthcare sites primarily for health professionals

Many of these sites are aimed at health professionals. They provide the best broad information on the growing field of evidence-based medicine. There are many more and these are just a few that we would highly recommend.

The Cochrane Database of Systematic Reviews

Type in 'Cochrane' and find the Cochrane Library. This is part of an international group called the Cochrane Collaboration. The Cochrane systematic reviews are the summaries of high-quality evidence about effective treatments that we discussed earlier in this book. The abstracts (akin to executive summaries) are available free to anyone and in some countries you can access the full version of the systematic reviews. Search the electronic Cochrane Library for a systematic review on your area of interest (for example, osteoarthritis)

Medline via 'PubMed'

If you type in 'PubMed' you'll find this free version of Medline that is run by the US National Library of Health. You can search for original articles in most medical journals here by typing in a keyword from the article's title and/or the authors surname or year of publication. All of the abstracts (executive summaries) are available free of charge and some of the complete articles are also linked.

Centre for Evidence-Based Medicine

This is a UK site aimed mainly at health professionals, but has useful background information on evidence-based medicine and links to relevant journals, including ones on evidence-based nursing and mental health.

Bandolier

This is a monthly journal produced in the UK which started in 1994 and features articles mainly on evidence-based primary care. They have a special website section about complementary and alternative medicine, the Oxford Pain Internet site, the Healthy Living site and the Migraine site, each of which features evidence summaries in these areas.

Users' Guide to the Medical Literature

This is available under subscription and is an interactive online tool for guiding clinicians in appraising evidence in their daily practice. It has been developed by the international 'Evidence-Based Medicine Working Group' who wrote a well-known series of articles for the *Journal of the American Medical Association* (*JAMA*) during the late 1990s and early 2000s. The checklists for appraising the quality of research evidence and for applying them in practice have been included in this interactive online version.

Evidence-based healthcare sites for consumers and healthcare providers

This list is by no means exhaustive. It merely highlights a few good quality resources to get you started.

Ottawa Decision Aid Inventory

This website has a list of decision aids to help weigh up the pros and cons of test and treatment options. Many of these are accessible free of charge. The site is managed by researchers and health professionals at the University of Ottawa.

Sydney Health Decision Group

This website was developed by University of Sydney researchers and also includes free online decision aids, pod-casts of radio programmes, clinical practice guidelines and hosts the chapter summaries and links for *Smart Health Choices.*

DISCERN

This contains a useful tool for evaluating the quality of health information for consumers and was developed by researchers in Oxford. We refer to it in Chapter 12 of this book.

DiPEx

This online UK resource of a broad range of patient stories was referred to in Chapter 9.

Informed Health Online

This resource originated from the Cochrane Collaboration and is now funded by the German government. It contains plain language summaries of many systematic reviews from the Cochrane Library. It also has other video and decision aid interactive resources.

Medline Plus

This is the consumer version of Medline and is managed by the US National Library of Medicine. It contains many useful factsheets and summaries of evidence in plain language.

National Center for Complementary and Alternative Medicine

Run by the US National Institutes of Health, it contains up-to-date summaries of research on Biologically Based Practices, Energy Medicine, Manipulative and Body-Based Practices, Mind-Body Medicine and Whole Medical Systems

Best Treatments

This is a plain English version of 'Clinical Evidence', a summary of evidence on common problems. It is produced by the *British Medical Journal* (*BMJ*) and is available free of charge in some countries only.

National Library for Health (UK)

The Clinical Knowledge Summaries provide a lot of evidence summaries on a range of topics, including patient information leaflets that can be downloaded. From the library's homepage you can also access Bandolier, the Cochrane Library, Patient.co.uk and NHS Direct.

Health Insite

This is the Australian Government's consumer website for health information and meets the kind of quality standards that we have discussed in this book.

General government health departments and other official organisations

We have included only a few main sites from the UK, the USA, Australia and New Zealand. For other country-specific sites you should search for your government health department.

The United Kingdom

National Health Service (NHS)

Information about health services, links to cancer screening and other programmes.

National Institute for Health and Clinical Excellence (NICE)

Guidance and advice on promoting health and preventing disease.

Australia

National Health and Medical Research Council (NHMRC)

An index of NHMRC publications for consumers and health professionals. They include clinical practice guidelines, and information booklets on a wide range of topics, such as child and elderly health, dentistry, drugs and poisons, infectious diseases and environmental health.

Department of Health and Ageing, Australian Government

Includes policies, health service information and links to specific programmes about national health priority areas, immunisation, screening programmes and medication.

New Zealand

New Zealand Guidelines Group

A wonderful evidence-based website of clinical guidelines for practitioners and consumers. It is particularly strong in cardiovascular disease prevention.

United States of America

Agency for Healthcare Research and Quality (US Department of Health and Human Services)

This contains guidelines and policies and has an extensive consumer and patient section.

Travel and vaccine advice – Centers for Disease Control and Prevention

General travel information and advice that is specific to country and individual travel itineraries can be accessed along with up-to-date bulletins about disease outbreaks and health alerts from around the world.

Cancer councils and specialist associations

Cancer councils are generally community-based organisations committed to preventing cancer and enhancing the quality of life for people with cancer and their families. They provide information, education and support, and also fund research and professional development. Specialist associations exist for many diseases, disorders and other conditions such as arthritis, diabetes and heart disease.

Media

There is an increasing number of resources that give a critical review of health stories mainly from the print media. As many TV and radio stories arise from the print releases, you will often find the stories that you are looking for on these sites. Once again, this list is not exhaustive but offers a few examples for your interest. We have included some news websites that will be ideal for testing your newly acquired 'smart health choice' skills.

Hitting the Headlines (UK)

MediaDoctor (Australia), MediaDoctor Canada and Health News Review (USA)

Provides critical reviews of the latest media reports in these countries. There are also public discussion sections and opportunities to rate most articles.

ABC Radio's The Health Report (Australia)

Provides access to summaries and transcripts of programmes.

The New York Times Health Section

Contains articles on recent health issues and research. Here you can test your skills after reading this book.

BBC Health Section

Contains articles on recent health issues and research. Here you can test your skills after reading this book.

Some books that you might find interesting

Marcia Angell, *The Truth About Drug Companies: How they deceive us and what to do about it.* Scribe Publications, 2005.
A former editor of the *New England Journal of Medicine* blows the lid on the influence of pharmaceutical companies upon research and clinical practice.)

Imogen Evans, Hazel Thornton, Iain Chalmers. *Testing Treatments – Better research for better healthcare.* London: The British Library, 2006.
Another book that takes a scientific approach to health-care decisions.

Atul Gawande. *Complications*: *A Surgeon's Notes on an Imperfect Science.* Sydney, Australia: Allen & Unwin, 2002.

An insider's well written account of the fallibility of medicine.

Muir Gray. *The Resourceful Patient:* www.resourcefulpatient.org.
Hard copies can be ordered from this website or the book can be
read online. It gives further tips on how to find and use good health
information.

Marion Morra, Eve Potts. *Choices,* 4th edn. (*Choices: The Most
Complete Sourcebook for Cancer Information*) (paperback). London:
Harper Collins, 2001.

Timothy B McCall. *Examining Your Doctor, A patient's guide to avoiding
harmful medical care.* New York: Carol Publishing Group, 1995.
A thoroughly researched book about how to obtain the best quality
health care. Written by a physician and oriented towards American
health care.

Ray Moynihan. *Too Much Medicine? The business of health – and its
risks for you.* Sydney: ABC Books, 1998.
By a journalist who makes a critical analysis of the forces driving
modern medicine, and how this can be to patients' detriment.

Ray Moynihan, Alan Cassels. *Selling Sickness: How drug companies are
turning us all into patients.* Allen & Unwin, 2005.
A critical examination of disease-mongering by pharmaceutical
companies and other vested interests.

Guy Maddern. *Questions You Should Ask Your Surgeon.* Sydney: Bay
Books, 1994.
An easy-to-read guide to choosing a surgeon.

Merrilyn Walton. *The Trouble with Medicine.* Sydney: Allen & Unwin,
1998.
Walton, now an academic, previously headed a statutory authority
that investigates patients' complaints in New South Wales. She
describes some of the issues that can lie behind poor clinical or
unethical medical practices.

John RA Duckworth. *The Official Doctor/Patient Handbook – A
consumer's guide to the medical profession.* UK: Harriman House
Publishing.

A book describing the different medical specialties, some medical jargon and how to find your way through the medical system. As it is written with the British medical system in mind, some aspects may not be applicable to all countries.

Miles Little. *Humane Medicine*. Cambridge: Cambridge University Press, 1995.
By a retired professor of surgery turned philosopher, this book presents a philosophical and ethical perspective on some of the challenges facing medicine.

Thomas J Moore. *Deadly Medicine: Why thousands of patients died in America's worst drug disaster*. New York: Simon & Shuster, 1995.
An account of how market forces, rather than valid research, influenced the introduction in the 1980s of drugs that were supposed to prevent deaths from heart rhythm abnormalities.

Louise B Russell. *Educated Guesses: Making policy about medical screening tests*. Berkeley, CA: California University Press, 1994.
A book about screening for prostate cancer, cholesterol and cervical cancer. Aimed at policy makers, but reasonably accessible to consumers.

Thomas Gilovich. *How We Know What Isn't So: The fallibility of human reason in everyday life*. New York: The Free Press, 1991.
A fascinating look at how people hold on to erroneous beliefs even in the face of evidence to the contrary. For everyone.

AK Dewdney. *200 per cent of Nothing – From 'percentage pumping' to 'irrational ratios'*.
For anyone with an interest in numbers and logic.

Larry Laudan. *The Book of Risks – Fascinating facts about the chances we take every day*. USA: John Wiley & Sons, Inc. 1994.
An easy to read, not very technical book that puts daily risks into perspective.

Andrew Moore and Henry McQuay. *Bandolier's Little Book of Making Sense of the Medical Evidence*. Oxford: Oxford University Press, 2006.

Written for health professionals but readable to others with an interest in learning more about evidence-based health care.

H Gilbert, M Welch. *Should I be tested for cancer? Maybe not and here's why.* Berkeley, CA: University of California Press.
A challenging look at weighing up the pros and cons of cancer screening and testing.

G Gigerenzer. *Reckoning with Risk. Learning to live with uncertainty.* London: Penguin, 2003.
A fascinating look at how we understand and live with chance and probabilities.

The following books are written for health professionals but may be accessible to those who want something heavy duty:

David M. Eddy. *Clinical Decision Making – from theory to practice.* USA: Jones & Bartlett.

Robert Fletcher, Suzanne Fletcher, Edward Wagner. *Clinical Epidemiology – The essentials.* Baltimore, MA: Williams & Wilkins, 1988.

JA Muir Gray. *Evidence-based Healthcare – How to make policy and management decisions.* London: Churchill Livingstone, 1997.

Bill Runciman, Alan Merry, Merrilyn Walton. *Safety and Ethics in Healthcare: A guide to getting it right.* Ashgate, 2007.

David Sackett, Scott Richardson, William Rosenberg, Brian Haynes. *Evidence-based Medicine – How to practice and teach EBM.* Oxford, UK: Elsevier, 2001.

Harold Sox, Marshal Blatt, Michael Higgins, Keith Marton. *Medical Decision Making.* USA: Butterworths, 1988.

AL Cochrane, *Effectiveness and efficiency – Random reflections on health services.* The Rock Carling Fellowship 1971. Cambridge: The Nuffield Provincial Hospitals Trust, 1972.

Glossary

Absolute risk reduction (ARR) or risk difference: the difference in the incidence of poor outcomes between the intervention group of a study and the control group. For example, if 20 per cent of people die in the intervention group and 30 per cent in the control group, the ARR is 10 per cent (30–20 per cent).

Abstract (of a study): a summary of the main features of a study. Major journals now use subheadings (similar to those in the main paper) to make it a structured abstract. These subheadings are, for example: introduction, methods, results and conclusions.

Adverse reaction: a side effect or unintended bad outcome of a treatment.

Anecdotal evidence: evidence that comes from an individual experience. This may be the experience of a person with an illness or the experience of a practitioner based on one or more patients outside a formal research study.

Benefit (of a health intervention): the extent to which one's lifespan is increased and/or quality of life improved

Bias: something that distorts the real effect in a study, so that the researchers get the wrong answer. The term does not suggest that the researchers are biased, but rather that sources of error can easily occur in studies.

Blinding and double-blinding: methods of preventing individuals, healthcare providers and those assessing outcome in a study from knowing whether the participant is in the experimental or control group.

Case–control study: involves selecting people who have the outcome of interest (cases), and a control group without the outcome of interest, and looking backwards in time to see if the groups were exposed to a supposed cause. These studies are not considered high-quality evidence unless the association is very strong; for example, case–control studies on lung cancer and smoking. Case–control studies are either population based or hospital based. The latter is the less reliable of the two.

Clinical practice guideline: a systematically developed statement designed to assist practitioner and patient to decide on appropriate care for specific clinical circumstances. Not all practice guidelines are based on the best available evidence.

Clinical trial: a study in which an intervention is being tested (see *Trial*).

Cochrane Collaboration: an international organisation that prepares, maintains and disseminates systematic reviews of the effects of healthcare. Publication is electronic. Abstracts are available free of charge on the internet.

Cohort study: an observational study that involves classifying people by their exposure to a study factor (for example, environment or lifestyle) of interest and following them over a period of time to see whether those exposed are more or less likely to develop disease than those not exposed.

Complementary medicine: any alternative or 'eastern' doctrine of healthcare. For example, naturopathy, homeopathy, reflexology, acupuncture, traditional Chinese medicine.

Confidence interval: even if studies are perfectly designed and carried out, the results may show variability because of the play of chance. A confidence interval covers the likely range of the true effect. For example, the result of a study may be that 40 per cent

(95 per cent confidence interval 30–50 per cent) of people are helped by a treatment. That means that we can be 95 per cent certain that the true effect is between 30 and 50 per cent.

Confounder: something that could explain an association between a study factor and outcome. For example, workers in a factory may get more lung cancer than those working elsewhere not because of their work but because they happen to be exposed to another known cause of lung cancer, cigarette smoking. In this example, smoking is the confounder and factory work may no longer be associated with lung cancer once the confounder has been taken into account.

Controlled trial: an intervention study in which a group given some intervention is compared with a control group.

Empirical evidence: evidence provided by experiments or observational studies rather than theory, assumptions or recall of single experiences.

Evidence-based medicine (healthcare): an approach to making health decisions that uses the best available evidence from good studies in combination with information from the patient.

Experimental study: see *Intervention study*.

Harm (of an intervention): the extent to which one's lifespan is shortened or one's quality of life deteriorates.

Incidence: the number of new cases of a disease in a given period of time as a proportion of the population.

Intervention: any therapy, surgical procedure, diagnostic or screening test or change in lifestyle or behaviour intended to have an effect on health.

Intervention study: an experimental study in which people are given an intervention to assess its effects. Examples are clinical trials, controlled trials and randomised controlled trials.

Lead time bias: a bias that occurs in the assessment of screening. As people who have been screened have their disease detected earlier, they live longer from the time of diagnosis, even if screening has no beneficial effects. This means that they have been given more years of disease rather than more years of life.

Medline: an electronic database of the titles and abstracts of many medical journals. A version called PubMed is available free of charge on the internet.

Meta-analysis: see *Systematic review*.

Number needed to treat (NNT): the number of people who must be treated to result in benefit in one person. It is the inverse of absolute risk reduction.

Observational study: a non-experimental study that examines the association between a study factor (for example, exposure or lifestyle) and outcome. Examples are cohort and case–control studies.

Odds ratio: a way of measuring relative risk.

Orthodox or mainstream medicine: conventional or 'western' doctrine of healthcare.

Outcome: any identified change in health status after a disease, an exposure to something or a preventive or therapeutic intervention. By comparing the outcomes of two experimental groups, one that receives the intervention and one that does not, the effect of an intervention can be assessed. Most often, the frequency of bad outcomes (that is, poor health or death) is measured.

Placebo: an inert treatment (or procedure); one that is not expected to have any pharmacological effect.

Placebo effect: a change caused by an expectation that the treatment or procedure will have an effect rather than directly by the treatment or procedure itself. The placebo effect is usually but not necessarily beneficial.

Post-test probability: the probability of having a disease after having a test. A positive test result will increase the probability of disease above the pre-test probability. A negative test result will decrease the probability of disease below the pre-test probability.

Practitioner: anyone who offers any form of healthcare in a professional capacity. For example, doctors, nurses, homeopaths, naturopaths, dentists, nutritionists, pharmacists, chiropractors, physiotherapists, occupational therapists, surgeons, veterinarians.

Pre-test probability: the probability of having a disease before having a test (see *Post-test probability*).

Prevalence: the total number of people who have the disease or condition at a particular time expressed as a proportion of the population.

Randomisation: allocation based on chance to either an intervention group or a control group of a study. This ensures that the outcomes in the groups are expected to be the same if the intervention has no effect.

Randomised controlled trial (RCT): a trial in which people are allocated randomly to either an intervention group or a control group.

Randomised trial: same as randomised controlled trial.

Recall bias: differences in the completeness or accuracy of recall of prior events, for example, mothers whose children died of leukaemia may be more likely to remember exposure of the unborn infant to X-rays than a control group of mothers.

Regression to the mean: many illnesses get better on their own and many abnormal findings become more normal on re-measurement in the absence of any intervention.

Relative risk (RR): the rate (risk) of poor outcomes in the intervention group divided by the rate of poor outcomes in the control group. For example, if the rate of poor outcomes is 20 per cent in the intervention group and 30 per cent in the control group, the relative risk is 0.67 (20 per cent divided by 30 per cent). The relative risk is 1 when the intervention has no effect, below 1 when it does good and above 1 when it does harm (see *Absolute risk reduction*).

Relative risk reduction (RRR): the extent to which the risk of a poor outcome is reduced by an intervention. In the example given in **Relative risk** (above), the relative risk reduction, expressed as a percentage, is 33 per cent (1.0 – 0.67 = 0.33) (see *Absolute risk reduction*).

Risk: the probability that an event will occur, for example, that an individual will die or become ill within a stated period of time.

Selection bias: error caused by systematic differences in characteristics between those who are selected and followed up in the intervention and control groups or the groups being compared in an observational study.

Sensitivity of a test: the probability of a positive test in people who have the disease of interest.

Specificity of a test: the probability of a negative test in people who don't have the disease of interest.

Systematic review: a review in which all relevant studies are identified and those of adequate quality selected. Results from adequate studies are usually pooled (meta-analysed) to give the best single estimate of effect.

Trial: an experiment or intervention study where a specific treatment or other intervention is 'tried' on a group of people; it is a synonym for clinical trial. Unless otherwise stated, a trial might not include a control group (see *Clinical trial*, *Controlled trial* and *Randomised controlled trial*).

After you read this book

As we pointed out at the start, we have designed this book in six parts to help you consider how health advice can improve your healthcare and, in fact, how it can be harmful. Some parts are more complex and detailed than others and you might have decided to skip these on first reading. However, as new health issues arise and you become more adept at using the skills that you have learnt here, you might want to re-visit relevant chapters and dip into some of those that you haven't yet looked at in depth.

The five 'smart health choices essential questions' in Chapter 5 are the core of this book and we urge you to use them and other tips from this book in making many of your own health decisions.

We hope that this book has given you the ability and confidence to begin to take control of your own health and make smarter health choices.

Index